"Seth Roberts, during a twenty-year bout of fiendish creativity, was willing to use his own body as a laboratory, and now has hit upon a weight-loss theory that just might benefit a few million people. This is what can happen when creative people ask smart questions, and have the relentless energy to follow through."

—*Stephen J. Dubner, coauthor of* Freakonomics

"In fact, it might benefit a few billion."

—*Dennis Prager, radio talk-show host*

"Instant willpower!"

—Woman's World

"Absurd, ridiculous, and remarkable. It is quite simply one of the most unusual weight-loss books ever written. . . . I have an inkling that Seth Roberts just might be onto something. *The Shangri-La Diet* is most certainly a paradigm-shifter of epic proportions."

—*Diet-Blog.com*

"Everything on the cover is literally true. You make one almost-subtle change, and you lose weight. . . . The first and only diet book that I've ever seen that really delivers."

—*CalorieLab.com*

"The Diet to End All Diets. It's like a diet pill in book form. No one need ever be fat again!"

—*Joyce Cohen,* New York Times *columnist and blogger (*Hunt Grunt*)*

"The strangest, easiest way to lose weight."

—*Kathy Sierra, blogger (*Creating Passionate Users*) and author of* Head First Java

The
SHANGRI-LA
DIET

The No Hunger

Eat Anything

Weight-Loss Plan

Seth Roberts, Ph.D.

A PERIGEE BOOK

A PERIGEE BOOK
Published by the Penguin Group
Penguin Group (USA) Inc.
375 Hudson Street, New York, New York 10014, USA

Penguin Group (Canada), 90 Eglinton Avenue East, Suite 700, Toronto, Ontario M4P 2Y3, Canada
(a division of Pearson Penguin Canada Inc.) · Penguin Books Ltd., 80 Strand, London
WC2R 0RL, England · Penguin Group Ireland, 25 St. Stephen's Green, Dublin 2, Ireland (a division of
Penguin Books Ltd.) · Penguin Group (Australia), 250 Camberwell Road, Camberwell, Victoria
3124, Australia (a division of Pearson Australia Group Pty. Ltd.) · Penguin Books India Pvt. Ltd., 11
Community Centre, Panchsheel Park, New Delhi—110 017, India · Penguin Group (NZ), 67 Apollo
Drive, Rosedale, North Shore 0745, Auckland, New Zealand (a division of Pearson New Zealand
Ltd.) · Penguin Books (South Africa) (Pty.) Ltd., 24 Sturdee Avenue, Rosebank, Johannesburg 2196,
South Africa

Penguin Books Ltd., Registered Offices: 80 Strand, London WC2R 0RL, England

While the author has made every effort to provide accurate telephone numbers and Internet addresses
at the time of publication, neither the publisher nor the author assumes any responsibility for errors,
or for changes that occur after publication. Further, the publisher does not have any control over and
does not assume any responsibility for author or third-party websites or their content.

PRINTING HISTORY
G. P. Putnam's Sons hardcover edition / April 2006
Perigee trade paperback edition / May 2007

Perigee trade paperback ISBN: 978-0-399-53316-7

The Library of Congress has cataloged the G. P. Putnam's Sons hardcover edition as follows:

Roberts, Seth Douglass, date.
    The Shangri-la diet: the no hunger, eat anything weight-loss plan/Seth Roberts.
    p.   cm.
    Includes bibliographical references and index.
    ISBN 0-399-15364-0
    1. Reducing diets.   2. Weight loss.   I. Title.
    RM222.2.R632   2006   2006041610
    613.2'5—dc22

PRINTED IN THE UNITED STATES OF AMERICA

10   9   8   7   6   5   4   3   2   1

PUBLISHER'S NOTE: Neither the publisher nor the author is engaged in rendering professional information, advice, or services to the individual reader. The ideas, procedures, and suggestions contained in this book are not intended as a substitute for consulting with your physician. All matters
regarding your health require medical supervision. In particular, excess weight can be associated with
"hidden" ailments, such as heart disease and diabetes, that should be medically determined before
undertaking a major change in your dietary habits. Neither the author nor the publisher shall be li-
able or responsible for any loss or damage allegedly arising from any information, advice, or suggestion in this book.

Most Perigee Books are available at special quantity discounts for bulk purchases for sales promo-
tions, premiums, fund-raising, or educational use. Special books, or book excerpts, can also be created to fit specific needs. For details, write: Special Markets, Penguin Group (USA) Inc., 375 Hudson
Street, New York, New York 10014.

To animal-learning researchers everywhere

CONTENTS

Let them gather all the food of these good years. . . . That food shall be a reserve for the land against the seven years of famine.

—GENESIS 41

Curiously enough, the immense dinner of the night before, which ought to have lasted me a week, made me hungrier than usual.

—*Love in a Cold Climate*

FOREWORD

The Shangri-La Diet, first published April 2006, came into a world not expecting it. There had been a *Freakonomics* column in the *New York Times* about my work and a website started by someone else devoted to the diet, but these did not change the fact that the book was unlike any other diet book on the market. It described a counterintuitive, strikingly simple new way to lose weight that had no obvious precedent. Drink fat to lose fat? Really?

Was the world ready for such a break with the past? Fortunately for me and anyone who wants to lose weight, the answer was: Part of the world.

The plainest evidence of the openness to this new idea in weight loss was the rapid growth of the Internet forums for the book (http://boards. shangriladiet.com). Nine months after the book came out, the forums have more than thirty thousand posts from more than two thousand people, and they continue to grow steadily.

Thousands of forum posts have shown that SLD worked much better than any other diet the person had tried. "It's a miracle," one poster explained, "because it's an easy, cheap, and painless solution to a very serious problem. What makes it a *bloody* miracle is the unexpectedness of it. . . . In my heart of hearts, I was sure I'd never be thin again."

Many of the posts describe how the diet has affected appetite ("my night snacking cravings are just gone") and eating behavior ("turning down chocolate," "only eating when I'm actually hungry"), confirming what the book describes.

Much of my professional life has involved statistics and data analysis; I was able to put these skills to good use because a poster in Texas named Rey Arbolay started and has maintained a special place on the forums for posting SLD weight-loss progress. To date, about one hundred people have provided data. This moved the evidence that the diet worked beyond a series of single cases. (For my analysis of this data, see "What to Expect," page 81.) As far as I know, such broad and detailed information is not widely available for any other weight-loss method.

On the other hand, forum posts also pointed out some weaknesses, limitations, and failures of SLD. The first version of the diet did not work for everyone, and some people lost weight only slowly. As these results came in (along with many more positive results), I began to feel as if I had an army of remarkably resourceful and dedicated people on my side. Slowly but surely, like a large group of workers pulling something heavy up a hill, the forum's posters have improved the diet. I had been studying weight control for more than fifteen years; in nine months the forums improved on the best I had been able to do. The updates in this edition of the book are mainly based on these improvements.

The improvements have taken many forms. Although the initial edition of the book placed equal emphasis on sugar water and flavorless oil, it soon became clear that oil was by far preferred. Many people had trouble drinking oil. A method for drinking oil easily was invented and tested (see page 66).

The abundance of support and assistance that forum members offered to anyone who posted results or asked a question helped many people try various alternatives until they found one that worked—thus educating all of us. Forum polls allowed a different kind of helpful comparison. Anyone could post a multiple-choice question and over the next few weeks many people would answer it. This gave new dieters a better idea of what to expect and helped them make better choices.

The biggest improvement to the diet came by e-mail. Gary Skaleski, a counselor in Wisconsin, remembered something from a high-school science class: If you hold your nose, an apple and an onion taste the same. He bought swimmer's nose clips and ate small amounts of food, such as a banana, while wearing them. This reduced his appetite quite effectively, especially because, unlike drinking olive oil, it gave him "that satisfying full-in-the-belly feeling." After nose-clipping ordinary food (eating it while wearing nose clips) worked for Gary and me and a few others, I posted the idea on the forums. Many people tried it and have found it effective. (See pages 94–96 for more on this "extra credit" weight-loss method.)

The abundance of gratitude expressed on the forums has been very satisfying, but forum posters have also given me something tangible and precious: better sleep. I started SLD using sugar water then switched to extra-light olive oil (ELOO) about three years ago. When the book was published, I drank ELOO every day. Reading the forums, however, I was struck by how often people reported better sleep. (About three-quarters of SLDers notice this, a forum poll showed.) Sleep is controlled by the brain, of course; could a few tablespoons per day of the right oil improve brain function? This was the tantalizing implication. It led me to study research on the effects of omega-3 (see pages 58–61), which suggested that, yes, 1 to 2 tablespoons a day of an omega-3-rich oil might indeed improve brain function. I switched from ELOO to refined walnut oil and flaxseed oil and found that my sleep, mental clarity, and balance all improved. Now I drink walnut oil and flaxseed oil every day. The improvements have continued (and the weight-control benefits have as well). Better sleep, mental clarity, and balance—what a gift! (Flaxseed oil has a strong flavor, so when I drink the flaxseed oil, I do so with my nose clipped shut.)

We live in a *Wisdom of Crowds* world where aggregation of information from many people is common, or at least a lot more common than ten years ago. Prediction markets, *Wikipedia*, and open-source software are three recent examples. The SLD forums are another example. They are tiny compared to, say, *Wikipedia*, but they go where these aggregating processes have not yet gone—into health improvement. They have improved a new way of losing weight; they have shown in great numerical detail what to expect; they have suggested that omega-3 can improve sleep. All this in nine months. What has happened on the SLD forums raises the real possibility that something like *Wikipedia* and open-source software—the high-quality product of thousands of talented people working together for free—will someday improve our health in many ways. It is a wonderful prospect. I hope this updated edition of *The Shangri-La Diet* does justice to what the SLD forums have accomplished so far.

Seth Roberts

Berkeley, California

January 2007

The
SHANGRI-LA
DIET

INTRODUCTION

Shangri-La? Odd name for a diet. Name of a spa, maybe. I chose it partly because Shangri-La, James Hilton's fictional Himalayan community, was a place of great peace and tranquility, and this diet puts people at peace with food. Within days after starting it, all sorts of food-related struggles (irresistible cravings, too many food-related thoughts, uncontrollable night eating) usually go away. (For examples, see "In Shangri-La," pages 84–91.) Another reason for the name was that Shangri-La was meant to be a near-perfect place and—not to boast—this is a diet with many advantages. It is simple, powerful, and does not require deprivation. It's almost as easy as taking a pill, and a hundred times safer and less expensive. I also liked the idea of naming a diet after an imaginary place.

Imaginary places are often full of novelty and hope—think Alice in Wonderland or Harry Potter. No harm in borrowing some of that.

Blog postings about the diet that appeared while I was writing it (see "The Blogosphere Tries It," pages 113–122) confirmed my choice of name. "Last week a neighbor dropped off a piece of chocolate cake and it actually went stale. I forgot it was there," wrote one dieter. "Unheard of." Many dieters expressed pleasure and amazement. "Ridiculously easy. And cheap. And effective. What hath God wrought?" wrote one of them. "I hardly believe it myself," wrote someone else in response to skepticism—someone for whom the diet was working. It was a little like being able to see the future: a glimpse of how the diet would be received.

How did such an unusual diet come to be? I think my secret weapon was that I combined three methods of investigation that had not been combined before. One was my scientific training, which made it easy for me to understand the relevant research literature. Another method I used was self-experimentation: I wanted to lose weight and tried many ways of doing so. The third method was to play reporter: to phone weight-control experts and ask them about their research. (I learned that experts were approachable in this way when I wrote for *Spy* magazine.) By themselves, none of these methods is unusual, but they are rarely, if ever, combined. For example, millions of people try various ways of losing weight, but few obesity researchers do (or at least they don't mention it): Self-experimentation is considered disreputable. Because I studied weight loss in a new way, it is more understandable that I reached surprising conclusions.

After a talk by a young scientist, Niels Bohr, the Danish physicist, said to him, "We are all agreed that your theory is crazy. The question that divides us is whether it is crazy enough to have a chance of being correct." That was a rather flashy way of putting it. In an essay in *Atomic Physics and Human Knowledge*, Bohr was more sober. "The common aim of all science," he wrote, is "the gradual removal of prejudices." It was another way of saying the same thing: The truth (that is, good science) may appear crazy at first because it does not fit our accepted views of how things work.

Everyone will agree that the Shangri-La diet contradicts accepted views about how to lose weight. In the 1980s, the mantra was *eat less fat*. Consumers were offered low-fat pizza, low-fat cookies, low-fat everything. The Shangri-La diet says you can lose weight by consuming *more* fat (in the form of flavorless oils). In the 1990s, the mantra became *eat fewer carbs*. The Shangri-La diet says you can lose weight by consuming *more* sugar, the worst carb of all. If Niels Bohr wanted to lose weight, I like to think he would try it.

1

WHY A CALORIE IS NOT A CALORIE

One of the guys said to the other, "What I don't understand is how a girl can eat a one-pound box of candy and gain 10 pounds."

—*The Daily Californian*

THE NOVELIST Vladimir Nabokov coined the term *doughnut truth* to mean "only the truth, and the whole truth, with a hole in the truth." This is a good description of what we have been told about weight loss by experts. What they've said isn't wrong, exactly, but it is seriously incomplete—and the missing information is very important if you want to lose weight easily and comfortably. The Shangri-La diet allows you to do just that because it's based on the whole truth—including the previously left-out "hole."

You've probably heard the phrase *a calorie is a*

calorie. Doctors say it to patients. Weight-loss experts say it to journalists. *A calorie is a calorie* is meant to convey the common belief that the only way to lose weight is to eat fewer calories than you burn. (A food's calorie value indicates how much energy you extract when you digest it. Like the mileage ratings of new cars, the calorie values of foods are measured under unrealistic conditions—but, like those mileage ratings, they're good for comparisons.) According to this idea, if a particular diet was successful it's because you ate fewer calories. The "calorie is a calorie" experts say that in order to lose weight you must put down your fork. Do whatever it takes to eat less. "Everything should be about portion size," said Marion Nestle, a professor of nutrition at New York University, in a radio interview. Anyone who says otherwise, they imply, who says that two foods with the same number of calories may have very different effects on your weight—well, that person is . . . confused.

It *is* true that in order to lose weight you must eat less or become more active—but it is *not* true that this has to be difficult. It is not even true that to lose weight you must *try* to eat less. In fact, you can lose weight by eating *more* of certain foods—and this book explains how. You will *add* foods to your diet and you won't have to stop eating anything. Unless you want to lose a large amount of weight (say, 60 pounds or more), you may not even need to make big changes in what you eat.

The Shangri-La diet is so different from previous diets and what you have been told about weight loss because it is based on a new theory of weight control, a theory supported by considerable scientific evidence.

More Is Easier Than Less

Early weight-loss diets demanded that you *subtract*: Cut calories by eating less. This prescription worked so rarely (everyone became too hungry!) that the message had to change. It became: *Eat less fat.* Cut out the ice cream, butter, French fries, hamburgers, and other high-fat foods, experts said, and the unwanted pounds will come off. This advice didn't work very well either.

The message became: *Eat fewer carbs.* Avoid almost all carbs (Atkins) or avoid "bad" carbs (Protein Power, Sugarbusters, South Beach), we were told, and you'll be healthier and slimmer. Bread, pasta, even apples and bananas were restricted or forbidden. Low-carb diets work modestly well, but they are not easy to follow ("I got tired of chicken and eggs," a friend said) and rarely produce as much weight loss as the dieter would like.

With the Shangri-La diet, weight loss happens because you *add*: You add certain foods to what you eat. These foods make you feel full and satisfied more easily; as a result, you eat less overall and lose weight. The foods you'll be adding are safe, cheap, and widely available. You don't have to give up anything. You don't need to *try* to eat less of any-thing or to pay close attention to how much you eat.

The Truth You Know

The Shangri-La diet is different from earlier diets because it is based on new ideas. One of them is that what you eat affects your weight in two ways—one that you already know all about, and one that's the missing hole in the whole dieting truth.

What you already know is that excess calories become fat. You've been told many times that your weight depends on how much you eat. If you eat more, you will weigh more. It's true that your body extracts energy (calories) from the food you eat, and if you consume more energy than you use most of the excess is stored as fat. From this point of view, it is true that a calorie is a calorie. It doesn't matter where the excess energy (calories) came from. It will become fat. As far as fat storage goes, 100 excess calories from raw carrots will have the same effect as 100 excess calories from banana cream pie. It is also true that to lose weight (fat), you must burn more calories than you eat. All this is true, but it is a doughnut truth.

The Missing Truth

Here is what you have not been told: Food also af-fects your weight by influencing what is called your body-weight *set point*, a term taken from engineering. Weight-control researchers have used it to mean the weight your body "wants" to be—the weight you are when you're not paying attention to how much you eat. Your set point may be quite a bit more than the weight you would choose or the weight that's healthy for you. In spite of the name, however, your set point is not fixed or constant. It is not your "natural weight," one unchanging magic number. Rather, your set point goes up and down, partly in response to what you eat.

By varying how hungry you are and how soon you feel full when you eat, your body-weight regulatory system pushes your weight close to your set point. Your body-weight set point is like the temperature to which a thermostat is set. My home thermostat, for example, is set to 68 degrees. The system "wants" the temperature to be 68 degrees at all times. If the temperature goes below 68 degrees, the system turns on a heater, which warms the house. When the temperature reaches 68 degrees, the heat goes off.

Your weight-regulation system controls your weight in a similar way. Let's say your body-weight set point is 180 pounds. If you weigh *less* than 180 pounds, you will be hungry and think about food. The bigger the gap between your set point and your weight, the more hungry you will be, the more you will think about food, and the more food it will take to feel full when you eat. It is nearly impossible to weigh much less than your set point for a long time—the hunger becomes unbearable.

If you weigh *more* than your set point of 180 pounds, you will not be hungry and will think much less about food. When you eat, you will feel full rapidly. (See the table for more details.)

The level of your set point depends on everything you have eaten for the last several months. Some foods are high-set-point foods; if you eat only these foods, your set point will be high. Some foods are low-set-point foods; if you eat only these foods, your set point will be low. (I'll explain why in later chapters.) Other foods are in between. Your set point depends on the *average* of what you have eaten for several months. When you eat a food that is low for you (lower than your average), your set

What's My Set Point?

IF YOU FEEL . . .	YOUR SET POINT IS . . .
Ravenous. Can't stop thinking about food. Dream about it. Nothing fills you up, even a large meal. Unhappy.	Your weight plus several pounds.
Hungry. Always feel like eating. Think about food every few minutes.	Your weight plus a pound or two.
Comfortable. Hungry sometimes. At mealtime, food looks good. You eat average amounts.	Close to your weight.
Full long after a meal. Forget to eat. Don't think about food. Not hungry until you start eating.	Your weight minus a pound or two.
Stuffed. Feel like you don't want to eat for days. Your favorite foods? No thanks. Never hungry.	Your weight minus several pounds.

point goes down slightly. When you eat a food that is high for you (higher than your average), your set point goes up slightly.

When a food lowers your set point, you will be less hungry than usual afterward. You may wait longer than usual before your next meal and you will tend to eat less than usual at your next meal. When a food raises your set point, you are more hungry than usual afterward, you may eat sooner than usual, and you will tend to eat more than usual at your next meal. The quote from Nancy Mitford's *Love in a Cold Climate* that opens this book (see page ix) is an example: The dinner raised the speaker's set point. It made her "hungrier than usual" at later meals.

By raising or lowering your set point, every food controls how much you eat *later*—how much you eat of *other* foods. By itself, a one-pound box of chocolates can increase your weight by no more than one pound. But if it raises your set point 10 pounds, it will cause you to eat more of *other* foods, enough to raise your weight 10 pounds. Your body always wants your weight to match your set point.

Diets and Your Set Point

Diets are not only about losing weight; they're also about how they make you feel. If you lose weight but feel hungry all the time, the diet is no success. You are very likely to regain the lost weight, sooner or later, in order to stop feeling hungry. This is why simply eating less doesn't work for long. You lose weight, true, but you gain hunger. Your hunger grows and eventually becomes unbearable.

Diets cause hunger when they lower your weight without lowering your set point. *The key to successful weight loss is to lower your set point.* When you lower your set point, you will lose weight without effort.

The Shangri-La diet lowers your set point because you eat *more* of certain foods—zero-set-point foods. These foods are so powerful that they will lower your set point no matter where it is. Because your set point will go down, you will feel less hungry than usual, you will eat less than usual, and you will lose weight—without any struggle at all. And without cutting anything out of your diet.

Your Set Point (Continued)

Let's go back to the thermostat analogy to understand more about your set point. A heating system with a thermostat has a set point: the temperature to which the thermostat is set. Just as the thermostat's set point is flexible (I can set it to 70 degrees, 60 degrees, and so on), so too is your body-weight set point.

To sum up, your home thermostat and your body's weight-regulation system have important similarities. Both have a set point. Both have a *flexible* set point.

There are also important differences:

- You can quickly change the thermostat's set point—by turning a dial. Your body-weight set point changes slowly, usually by no more than a few pounds per week.

- Your body-weight set point is designed to be sensitive to the price of energy (calories). When energy is cheap—that is, when calories are abundant—your body-weight set point goes up. Hundreds of thousands of years ago, when our body-weight regulation system evolved, this strategy made sense. Food was often scarce, so when it was abundant it made sense to eat more than usual and store the excess as fat. When food was scarce, it made sense to use the stored energy and lose weight. However, our current conditions are drastically different from the conditions thousands of years ago. Food is now abundant all the time. As a result, this pricing/storage mechanism no longer works well. Your system decides (correctly) that food is abundant and thus raises your set point to increase the amount of energy you have stored— but the lean years never come. The Shangri-La diet tricks your system into thinking food is *scarce*, thus solving the problem. Your home thermostat is simpler: It isn't sensitive to the price of energy (electricity, natural gas, heating oil). It's not sensitive to outside conditions in any way.

- Most home thermostat systems are "all or none." Either the heat source is on (when the actual temperature is lower than the thermostat temperature) or off (when it's not). In contrast, your body-weight regulation system varies the strength of the push toward set point (hunger) according to how much difference there is between your actual weight and your set point. A small difference causes a little hunger. A big difference causes great hunger.

- To push a cold room (for example, one that's 60 degrees) toward the set point temperature (70 degrees), a home-temperature system will do just one thing: turn on the heat. In contrast, your body-weight regulatory system will cause at least three changes if your actual weight (150 pounds) is less than your set-point weight (155 pounds): You will feel more hungry than usual; you will think about food more often; and when you eat, it will take more food to make you feel full.

Systems with set points, bless them, are *set and forget*: Once the set point is in the right place, no further action is necessary. Once you have set your home's thermostat to the right temperature, you can forget about it. It will turn the heat on and off appropriately. Likewise, when you understand how to lower your body-weight set point, that is all you will need to know about losing weight. After you lower your set point, you will not need to think more about it. Your brain will turn hunger on and off (mostly off) in such a way that you will lose weight without struggle. Without counting calories. Without carefully choosing what to eat. Without going hungry.

How Does My Set Point Control My Weight?

If you are like most people, your body-weight set point is always close to your actual weight— sometimes slightly above, sometimes a bit below, but never far away. Your weight-regulation system keeps your weight close to your set point the way a driver keeps a car in its lane: by making many small adjustments. When your weight is slightly below your set point, you become a little more hungry than usual and it takes a little more food to feel full. When your weight is slightly above your set point, you feel slightly less hungry than usual and it takes a little less food to feel full. These changes in appetite are so small and frequent that we usually don't notice them.

If you follow the advice in this book, however, you should be able to move your set point well below your current weight—quite possibly farther below your weight than it has ever been before. Once your set point is lowered by simply adding certain foods to what you normally eat, you will be able to keep it there easily, without conscious effort. When your body-weight set point is lowered, you'll notice the following changes:

1. *You will be less hungry between meals.* You will feel less mental pressure to eat. It will be easier to avoid snacking. You'll think about food less often. If you're in the habit of eating late at night, you'll likely no longer want to.

2. *During a meal, you will feel full faster.* When you eat, it will take less food to make you feel full—to reach the point where you want to stop eating—so you will eat less. If your body-weight set point is below your actual weight, you will feel full sooner than if your set point is above your weight. In other words, when you change your body-weight set point to a significantly lower weight (by following the Shangri-La diet), you'll eat the same food and enjoy the same tastes, but you won't need to eat as much food in order to feel satisfied.

These two changes usually happen within days of starting the Shangri-La diet. They will be the first signs that the diet is working.

Some Flavors Are More Fattening Than Others

One of the most unusual features of the Shangri-La diet is its emphasis on flavor. The reason for this emphasis is that *the flavor of a food controls how it affects your set point.*

We are born liking sweet foods and salty foods,

but most flavors, such as the flavor of spinach, we learn to like—as parents know. Much of this learning is associative: We come to like a flavor when we associate it with calories. As a flavor becomes better associated with calories, it tastes better. Coke, the soft drink, is a good example. A Japanese cookbook author named Gaku Homma had his first taste of Coke when he was old enough to remember it. He later wrote it tasted "like medicine." A friend of mine had his first taste of Coke when he was seven or eight. It didn't taste good. *What was the fuss about?* he wondered. In both cases, the Coke did not taste good because the flavor had not yet become associated with calories. Because Coke contains calories, as you drink it again and again the flavor-calorie association becomes stronger and stronger and the flavor tastes better and better. Here is how a restaurant critic described his reaction to cilantro: "First put off by the leaves' flavor, after repeated exposure I grew to anticipate their taste. Then welcomed it. Then craved it." His reaction changed because he ate the cilantro with food (calories). Had he eaten it alone, his initial negative reaction would have persisted.

Flavor-calorie associations are important because they influence your set point. A food with a strong flavor-calorie association will raise your set point; a food with a weak flavor-calorie association will lower your set point; a food with *no* flavor-calorie association will lower your set point a lot.

Foods That Lower Your Set Point

Once you realize that lowering your set point is the key to losing weight, all you need to do to begin the Shangri-La program is eat foods that lower your set point.

If we rate foods on a scale from 0 to 10, where a food ranked at 0 pushes your set point toward zero (skinny) and food ranked at 10 pushes your set point toward a very high value (obese), we might say that raw vegetables have a value of 4, and junk food a value of 10. (Later, I'll explain why junk food pushes your set point very high, and the reason may surprise you.) If you eat only junk food (value of 10), your set point will be much higher than if you eat only raw vegetables (value of 4). Suppose you eat only junk food but then add raw vegetables to your diet. This will lower your set point, because you are adding 4's to a diet that otherwise is all 10's, and cause you to lose weight.

On your old diet, you ate foods that were 10, 10, 10, 10, 10; the average value of your diet is 10.

On your new diet, you added some lower-valued foods: 10, 10, 10, 10, 10, plus 4, 4. Now the average value of your diet is less than 10, so your set point will drop.

The Shangri-La diet is based on the discovery that there are foods far more powerful than raw vegetables at lowering your set point. If raw vegetables are 4, the foods at the heart of the Shangri-La diet are 0. Even small amounts of them will lower your set point significantly. Here is one of these set-point-lowering foods:

Extra-light olive oil. Extra-light olive oil has almost no flavor (the opposite of extra-virgin olive oil, which has a strong flavor). Swallowing a small amount of extra-light olive oil is very close to eating a food with no flavor, which, again, lowers your set point and helps you lose weight.

Even in amounts as small as a few hundred calories per day, this food has potent weight-loss effects. In later chapters we'll talk much more about this food, similar foods, and their benefits. What I hope you've learned at this point is that weight loss can be achieved in a surprising new way. While you probably haven't heard of this new method before, it's simple, easy to adopt, and perfectly consistent with a healthy diet. You don't need to stop eating anything. You don't need to stop eating hamburgers or desserts or bread, or, for that matter, any of the healthier choices you make. If you want to lose a great deal of weight, you may need to vary the *flavors* of your food—the flavor of your hamburgers, for example. Chapter 6, "Extra Credit: Eight More Ways to Lose Weight," is about how to apply the new ideas in other ways.

How much of these foods you will need to eat each day will depend on how much weight you want to lose, but you may need to eat as little as 200 calories a day or less of these Shangri-La set-point-lowering foods. When your set point becomes lower than your actual weight, you'll be less hungry throughout the day. When you eat, you will feel satisfied sooner. You will lose weight until your weight reaches your new, lower set point. And at that point, your hunger will return to normal levels and you will stop losing weight.

2

THE CASE OF THE MISSING APPETITE

*This new, $3 billion-a-year industry was aimed
squarely at the age-old pursuit of getting
thin while eating whatever you want,
which, of course, never works.*

—*The Washington Post* (2005),
DESCRIBING THE LOW-CARB FOOD INDUSTRY

INTRODUCTORY Psychology was the first class I taught when I became a professor. I decided to include a lecture on weight control—not a typical Psych 1 topic, but it interested me. It was an intellectual interest, not a practical one: I was thin and ate whatever I wanted. I read a stack of scientific articles to figure out what to say. Most of them were about rat experiments that had studied the effect of dietary changes on weight. I liked reading about rat experiments. In graduate school, I had done quite a few of them, although not in the area of weight control. My doctoral dissertation was about how rats measure time.

Ten years later, I was no longer thin. The scale read 200 pounds. I am five foot ten, so my BMI (body mass index) was 29 (overweight). I had lectured on weight control many times and had given my students advice based on the scientific papers I had read. Now I took my own advice and started eating less-processed food—oranges instead of orange juice, for example. The dietary change worked: I easily lost about ten pounds. This was intriguing. Maybe reading about all those rat experiments had taught me something useful.

I continued to read scientific papers about weight control. At one point, I planned to write a popular book based on my Psych 1 lectures. While doing research for the book (never finished), I spoke to Dr. Israel Ramirez, a research scientist at the Monell Chemical Senses Institute in Philadelphia. He sent me a stack of reprints of his scientific papers, and one of them led me to think of a new theory of weight control. (For more about Ramirez's research, see the Appendix, "The Science Behind the Theory Behind the Diet," pages 141–158) The theory, which I describe in the next chapter, helped me find two new ways of losing weight: eating food with a low glycemic index (I lost six pounds) and eating sushi (I lost thirteen pounds). This was excellent evidence that there was a lot of truth to it.

I never stopped eating less-processed food, and

never regained the weight I had lost that way. I never stopped eating food with a low glycemic index and never regained that lost weight either. I did stop eating sushi after a month or so and regained *that* lost weight. At this point, I weighed about 185 pounds (BMI 26, still overweight), definitely too much. Like a billion other people, I would have liked to lose weight but could not. Unlike them, however, I had a seriously good theory of weight control—a theory that had actually worked, in the sense that it had helped me lose weight. My situation puzzled me. If I truly understood weight control, shouldn't I be able to choose my weight? If you understand how something works, shouldn't you be able to fix it? I was unable to see the flaw in this argument, which seemed to imply there was something wrong with my theory. But I couldn't find anything wrong with it.

French Sodas Expand My Theory

In 2000, I went to Paris in order to get a cheap flight to Croatia to visit a friend. Paris being Paris, I stayed a week.

I love French food. My first meal in Paris, at a bistro, was delicious. After that meal, however, I lost my appetite. For most of the rest of my visit, I had to force myself to eat. Big disappointment!

Why? I wondered. I wasn't sick or depressed or anxious. I wasn't taking any medication. I was walking many miles per day, wandering around the city. Life was normal, for a vacation—I just didn't feel like eating. Usually I ate a lot.

As I explained in Chapter 1, "Why a Calorie Is Not a Calorie," my weight-control theory emphasizes that the relationship between your set point and your actual weight determines how hungry you are at any given moment. If your set point is *above* your weight, you will be hungry. If your set point is *below* your weight, you will not be hungry. Total loss of appetite, according to my theory, meant that my set point was well below my weight (see table, "What's My Set Point?," on page 10). I had plenty of time on my walks to think about what might have caused this.

I had never before lost my appetite so completely, so the cause was probably something unusual. Not Paris: I had visited Paris and other foreign cities without losing my appetite. My theory said that food controls the set point. So I focused on food: What unusual food had I eaten?

The bistro meal hadn't been unusual. But there *was* something different. It was June and very hot. To cool off, I had drunk a few sugar-sweetened soft drinks each day for several days. This was unusual—in fact, unprecedented. At home I never drank sodas with sugar; I always drank diet sodas. In Paris, I wanted to try drinks not available at home, but the new sodas I encountered didn't have diet versions. I had been forced to drink sodas with sugar.

These sodas had unfamiliar flavors. Their flavors were not yet associated with calories. According to my theory, as Chapter 1 said, *a food with no flavor-calorie association will lower your set point a lot*. This made me suspect the sodas.

If my theory was wrong, to focus on soft drinks was absurd. In Paris, I surely lost weight—that's what happens when you skip meal after meal. Almost everyone thinks sugar-sweetened soft drinks cause weight *gain*. But my theory said that only *familiar* sugar-sweetened soft drinks cause weight gain (by raising the set point); *unfamiliar* ones should cause weight *loss* because they lower the set point. If my theory was right, focusing on the French soft drinks made sense.

Fructose and the Flavor–Calorie Association

When I got home, I wanted to test the idea that it was the new soft drinks that had spoiled my appetite. One test would be to drink new-flavored soft drinks and see what happened. But this would be hard to sustain: I would run out of new flavors. Another test would be to drink soft drinks with *no* flavor. With no flavor, no flavor–calorie association can form. I couldn't avoid the familiar flavor of sweetness—the drinks had to contain calories—but maybe sweetness had little effect.

The test I chose was to drink fructose-sweetened water: water with nothing but fructose. Table sugar is sucrose. Fructose is a somewhat different sugar found in honey and fruit. It looks the same as sucrose but is slightly sweeter. I used fructose instead of sucrose because fructose is digested more slowly. (Eventually I decided that the difficulties of obtaining fructose outweighed its advantages, at least for most people, and I now suggest that people use sucrose as part of the Shangri-La diet.)

I drank the fructose water "unflavored"—with nothing but fructose—to avoid forming flavor–calorie associations. Had I added lemon juice, for example, a lemon flavor–calorie association might have formed.

The fructose water caused an astonishing loss of appetite. This was clear within hours. (I started with a dose that in retrospect was much larger than necessary. With a better, lower dose, it can take longer to notice the loss of appetite.) I ate much less than usual and lost weight fast. Fructose water suppressed my appetite much more than I expected. I halved my daily intake of fructose several times over the next few weeks, yet my appetite did not return. I continued to lose weight quickly, more than two pounds per week. I simply wasn't hungry, just like in Paris. It really had been the sodas.

This was stunning. There was no precedent anywhere—not in the research literature, not in my previous self-experimentation, not in any anecdote I had ever heard—for such a small change (a few hundred calories per day) causing so much weight loss. It was much easier than any other weight-loss method I knew of. I wasn't trying to eat less (classic advice) or eat within limits (Weight Watchers) or count calories (many diets) or avoid something (Atkins, South Beach, Zone, Protein Power) or be more active (classic advice). The fructose water seemed so powerful that it appeared that I could weigh whatever I wanted. I started at 185 pounds. I decided to stop at 150 pounds, a nice round number.

I drank a small amount of fructose water every day, adjusting the quantity up and down to find a level that left me with a little bit of hunger but not a lot. Some hunger was better than none because hunger made food taste better and, of course, I still needed to eat. I ate about one meal every two days. I was never unpleasantly hungry. Sometimes I wasn't hungry enough (as in Paris). A few times I stopped the fructose water for a few days in order to increase how hungry I felt—possibly a weight-loss first.

The weight loss wasn't completely painless. It was boring to eat so little. (Slower weight loss might have solved this problem.) I often just wanted taste, not calories: I started drinking several cups of tea each day and chewing gum. I began to love super-market samples: small portions, lots of taste. I also started seeking food that was crunchy (apples, crackers, nuts, popcorn) or chewy (gum, beef jerky, dried mango). This desire for crunchy and chewy foods was new.

I reached 150 pounds in three months (see Figure 1, page 28). "Are you dying?" a colleague asked. "Don't lose any more weight," said another

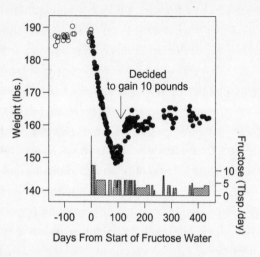

Figure 1. Weight loss from fructose water. The shaded area at the bottom indicates how much fructose I drank each day.

coworker. I bought new clothes. I had my belt shortened. To stay at 150, to stop losing weight, I reduced my fructose intake. I wanted my appetite back, but I didn't want to start gaining weight. The appropriate level for me turned out to be about 3 tablespoons of fructose (150 calories) per day. Had I stopped drinking fructose altogether, I would have slowly regained the lost weight (as others do when they stop the diet). At 150 pounds, friends gently told me I looked too thin. I took their word for it and intentionally gained ten pounds.

Why did fructose water work so well? My theory had led me to this surprising discovery—so the theory surely had a lot of truth to it—but it didn't fully explain the weight loss. My theory made a prediction: *Eating calories without flavor will lower your set point.* If you consumed all of your food without any flavor, the theory said, your set point would go close to zero (almost no body fat). Something like this seems to happen in hospitals, where some patients receive all nutrition, including calories, intravenously—without any flavor, in other words. They often lose a great deal of weight and become very thin without becoming hungry. I saw a mild example of this phenomenon recently. The mother of a friend of mine spent a few days in the hospital, where she was fed intravenously. Her appetite vanished, and remained very low for several days after she left the hospital. My explanation is that due to intravenous feeding, her set point dropped quite a bit while she was in the hospital.

However, unflavored fructose water *does* have flavor: It is sweet. To explain its weight-loss potency, I had to assume that sweetness is a kind of "invisible" flavor that does not become associated with calories. This was a reasonable assumption. As a flavor becomes associated with calories, it tastes better. That's why the restaurant critic mentioned in Chapter 1 liked the taste of cilantro more and more. Sweetness, however, tastes good regardless of experience; young children naturally like sweet things. Another striking difference between sweetness and other flavors is that sweet things taste less good when you are hungry. "There is something unpleasant or aversive about sweetness when food deprivation is high," wrote Dr. Elizabeth Capaldi, a professor of psychology at the University of Florida, Gainesville, based on her research. These differences between sweetness and other flavors made it more reasonable to assume that sweetness alone did not become associated with calories (and so did not raise the set point).

Fear No Food

I stayed in the 160s—a 20-pound weight loss—without difficulty. Drinking 100 to 200 calories a day of fructose water to keep my weight in check worked well. After about two years of this, a friend pointed out that a type of olive oil, called *extra-light*, has essentially no flavor. The flavor of olive oil, if any, comes from "impurities" (molecules other than fat). Extra-virgin or virgin olive oil has a greenish color and strong taste. Extra-light olive oil (also called *pure* and *extra-light-tasting*), however, is pure fat with no flavor and no greenish tint. *Extra-light* refers to flavor, not calories. Extra-light olive oil—ELOO, I'll call it—has the same number of calories per tablespoon as other olive oils, such as extra-virgin. They all contain about 120 calories per tablespoon. My friend understood that my theory predicted that the most potent weight-loss foods provided calories without flavor. Fructose water did this because of a special wrinkle: Sweetness didn't count. ELOO was another way. According to my theory, 100 calories of ELOO should have the same effect as 100 calories of fructose water.

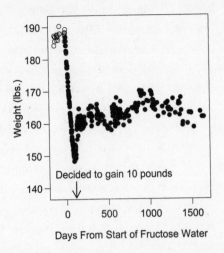

Figure 2. Long-term effects of fructose water and extra-light olive oil.

I tested this prediction. I stopped drinking fructose water and started swallowing the same caloric amount of ELOO, about 1 tablespoon per day. I found that the prediction was right: ELOO was roughly as effective per calorie as fructose water. I stayed at the same weight. Fructose water had pushed my set point down to a certain level and kept it there; the same calorie amount of ELOO also kept it there. Figure 2, on this page, shows that I have stayed close to my chosen weight for five years.

ELOO had two advantages over fructose (and sucrose) water. First, it took less time. A day's worth could be consumed in seconds. No preparation was needed, unlike sugar water. Second, it was probably healthier than sugar water. Olive oil is a staple of the Mediterranean diet, eaten by Italians, Greeks, and Cretans, groups of people who generally enjoy long lives and have low rates of heart disease. Surveys have found that people who consume more polyunsaturated fats, including olive oil, are in better health than those who consume less. Evidence for benefits of sucrose or fructose is harder to find.

For a few years, I drank only ELOO and didn't use fructose water. Eventually I resumed drinking fructose water as well, because in small amounts it is pleasant. Then I switched from fructose water to sucrose (regular table sugar) water because sucrose is much more available. ("Free in every restaurant in America," a friend of mine likes to say.) Now I drink both: ELOO or some other flavorless oil at home, sucrose water when I'm away from home. I don't measure the amounts. If I have gained a few pounds, I drink more. If I have become too thin, I drink less.

Even when my weight was constant (in the 160s), I continued to eat much less than I had eaten when my weight was in the 180s. My metabolism had slowed down. Experiments had shown this—when you lose weight, your metabolism slows down—but their results hadn't prepared me for the size of the reduction. Before losing weight, I ate two big meals per day. After losing weight, I ate one meal per day and a few snacks. In spite of eating many fewer calories each day, I neither lost weight nor felt hungry. The time savings was wonderful. The conventional benefit of weight loss is better health: Your risk of major illnesses (diabetes, heart disease, etc.) supposedly goes down and you live longer. But it would take many years of extra life to produce the free time I save by eating one less meal per day. Because I was eating much less, I was also spending much less money on food—about half of what I had previously spent.

"Free at last," spoken softly, was how I felt. Before weight loss, I had avoided many foods I liked because I knew they would cause me to gain weight. After weight loss, with the power of fructose or sucrose or ELOO behind me, I ate whatever I wanted, in moderation. When it came to desserts, jam, pasta, bread, cookies, and other baked goods, I ate small amounts, which were plenty. Restaurant portions looked huge. Above all, I could *relax*: If something was fattening, I could simply drink more sugar water the next day. Not only could I eat any-thing, I could also eat nothing—skip any meal—and feel fine. On a long flight, for example, if I didn't like the airplane food, I simply didn't eat it. Because I ate much less, I was happy to pay much more per meal. Food became less a necessity and more a treat. I was careful to get good nutrition (fruits, veg-etables, whole grains, vitamins, and minerals) every day.

My Eureka Moment

According to *New Yorker* writer Malcolm Gladwell, diet books "have an unspoken set of narrative rules and conventions," which include "the Eureka

Moment, when the author explains how he stumbled on the radical truth that inspired his diet." I too had a Eureka Moment, but it was not the sugar-water discovery.

It happened long before that: when I discovered that the weight-loss advice I had been giving my students actually worked. One conclusion in my lecture on weight control was that *the better food tastes, the more fattening it is*. What makes food taste good? Well, processing helps. Much of what we do to food improves the taste. This suggested that less-processed food—food closer to its natural state—would be less good tasting and therefore less fattening. I tested this prediction. I ate less-processed food: oranges instead of orange juice, brown rice instead of white rice or pasta, simple home-cooked food instead of take-out or deli food. I stopped eating baked goods, including bread. For the first few days, the new food seemed bland and dull. Within a week, however, I came to enjoy it and found my former food unappetizing.

As mentioned earlier, it worked. I lost ten pounds in eight weeks (see Figure 3, page 35). Apart from the modest difficulty involved in changing what I ate, it was effortless. For a while I felt less hungry than usual, so I ate less than usual and thereby lost weight. I never regained the lost weight. I never missed the food I stopped eating. Even now, fifteen years later, I still dislike orange juice and scones. The consensus among weight-loss experts has been that it is nearly impossible to lose weight

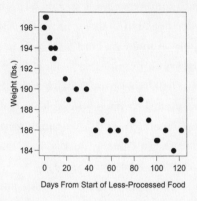

Figure 3. Weight loss when I started eating less-processed food—oranges instead of orange juice, for example.

and keep it off. "Weight loss is not for the faint-hearted," said Dr. Thomas Wadden, director of the Weight and Eating Disorders Program at the University of Pennsylvania, in 2005. But I had lost weight easily.

The "radical truth" that inspired my diet was not that eating less-processed food caused me to lose weight. That was just an interesting truth. The radical truth was how easy it had been to learn that interesting truth. I could not explain why my dietary change had caused weight loss. But I realized *I might be able to find out by studying myself.* In a world where a typical weight-loss study costs hundreds of thousands of dollars, takes several years, and is done by a team of scientists who have devoted their professional lives to the subject, to believe that someone like me—basically ignorant, with no credentials in physiology or nutrition—

could learn something important at no cost in a few months *was* radical. Self-experimentation has a long history in medicine, but it has almost always been used to show rather than to find. For example, Barry Marshall, winner of the 2005 Nobel Prize in Medicine, used his own body to show the truth of an idea about ulcers. The self-experimentation came long after the idea. My notion was that self-experimentation could *give* me ideas.

That is what happened. My weight-control theory was initially inspired by some rat experiments done by Israel Ramirez (see Appendix). But I came to believe the theory because it helped me find new ways of losing weight. When I lost my appetite in Paris, I believed my theory strongly enough to test the hypothesis that it suggested: that my loss of appetite was due to drinking sodas with unfamiliar flavors. And that hypothesis—which would strike most people, including most obesity researchers, as absurd—turned out to be correct.

〜 **Never This Thin**

ANDREA B., a forty-five-year-old computer operator in Souderton, Pennsylvania, was five feet eight inches tall and weighed 174 pounds (BMI = 26) when she learned about SLD in May 2006 from the *Dennis Prager Show*. She started it the same day. She wanted to lose ten pounds to fit into her summer clothes. Her eating habits puzzled her. "I am a reasonable, rational woman," she posted on the SLD forums. "I could never understand why I could not control my sometimes constant snacking. I never felt I was an emotional eater but I just felt compelled to be munching on something most times of the day."

SLD changed that. She started with 1.5 tablespoons of ELOO twice a day (= 3 tablespoons a day). During the first few days it took willpower to avoid eating during the two-hour window (see page 63), but after that it was effortless. After three or four days, she noticed she was getting full faster. After several months she posted this:

Within 4 days [of starting SLD] the snacking demons stopped and I didn't much think about food. My relationship to food was totally changed. I was AMAZED to say the least. I ate three meals (smaller than I used to eat) a day and an occasional snack.... My weight came off slowly but surely. One to two lbs a week average. Sometimes none. Sometimes 3 lbs. I went 2 or 3 weeks sometimes and didn't lose any. Then the weight loss would start again. I didn't concern myself with what I ate—I just ate what I felt like eating. If that was ice cream I ate it (amazingly I only wanted a small amount).

She had hoped to reach 164 pounds, but it was so easy that by October 2006 she had reached 140 pounds ("!!!!!!!!"). This was staggering: "I've never been this thin in my life." Another benefit, she says, is that "I used to get headaches before my period. At least 2 times/month. I don't get them anymore." She lost the weight without any change in exercise or activity. For her job she lifts lots of boxes. She walks a few miles twice a week and plays golf once a week.

After reaching 140, she stopped the ELOO out of curiosity. After three weeks off, "My eating has increased somewhat," she posted, "and I'm starting to feel a little bingey again." She resumed the ELOO. One tablespoon a day was not quite enough to keep her from gaining weight, she found; two tablespoons per day has worked fine.

What did she learn from the SLD forums? Patience. "I learned that weight loss was slow, that if your weight went up a little it wasn't any big deal because it would go down again. Knowing that helped when I went 2 weeks and didn't lose any-

thing." SLD is not really a diet, she says, "It's something extra you do to control your eating. . . . I didn't
feel like I had to decrease my calories to a low level;
my natural eating went down to a level that made
me lose weight."

3

A NEW THEORY OF WEIGHT CONTROL

This chapter explains the theory behind the diet. The theory doesn't merely explain why the diet works; it actually helped me discover it. After calorielab.com posted a long and skeptical account of this diet, someone commented, "I have been using the Shangri-La diet now for almost a month, and it works beautifully. . . . Who cares why?" Well, yes, not everyone cares. You don't need to understand the theory to do well with the diet. But I think some readers will want to. Maybe it will help *you* discover new ways of losing weight.

The theory consists of several interlocking ideas, which I will explain one by one.

Idea 1. Your weight is regulated by a system with a set point.

As Chapter 1, "Why a Calorie Is Not a Calorie," discussed, your body's weight-control system resembles a thermostat-controlled heating system. Just as a thermostat-controlled heating system has a set-point temperature that it tries to maintain, your body's weight-control system has a set-point *weight* that it tries to maintain. The Appendix, "The Science Behind the Theory Behind the Diet," describes some of the evidence for this idea.

The name *set point* may be confusing because the set point is *not* fixed or "set"; it may help to remember that the temperature to which a thermostat is set is not fixed either. *Set point* is just one of those terms whose meaning is quite different from the sum of its parts.

Idea 2. When your actual weight falls below your set point, your system makes you more hungry and increases how much food it takes to make you feel full.

When a thermostat detects that the room temperature is lower than the set point, it turns on the heat to warm up the room. Turning on the heat pushes the temperature back up toward the set point. When the temperature reaches the set point, the heat is turned off. When your body-weight regulatory system detects that you have less fat on your body than your set point, it makes you more hungry than usual between meals and increases how much food you need to eat to feel full. (There are other changes too, but these are the most obvious.) These changes cause you to eat more than usual and gain weight—pushing your weight back up toward your set point. As your weight gets closer to your set point, your hunger goes down.

Idea 3. Between meals, your set point goes down.

When you are not eating, your set point slowly goes down. The rate of decline varies widely (see Idea 4), but a very rough estimate is a half pound per day. (When you don't eat, your weight goes down too, of course, as you burn fat. Your weight goes down faster than your set point. That is why not eating causes hunger—and why diets that deprive you of food don't work.)

Idea 4. The higher your set point, the faster it goes down between meals.

If your set point is very high (you are obese), it may decrease between meals at the rate of one pound per day. If your set point is quite low (you are thin), it will decrease much more slowly—perhaps a quarter pound per day.

Idea 5. Eating flavors that are associated with calories raises your set point.

When you eat something with a calorie-associated flavor, your set point goes up. Any familiar food with calories (apple, bread, salmon) will do this.

Ideas 3 and 5 together imply that your set point is always going up and down: up at a meal (Idea 5), down between meals (Idea 3), up at a meal, down, etc. Figure 4, below, shows this oscillation.

Your set point will stay roughly the same—going up and down around the same value—only if the amount that food raises your set point *at* meals equals the amount that your set point goes down *between* meals. The chances are very good that right now this is true: The food you eat raises your set point by the same amount that it declines between meals. This keeps your set point stable—and therefore keeps your weight stable. (Your weight is always close to your set point.) The Shangri-La diet causes weight loss because it reduces how much your food increases your set point each day—you get the same number of calories but your set point goes up less. The result is that your current set point—and therefore your current weight—become unsustainable. Your set point will slowly fall until increase and decrease are back in balance.

For example, suppose your food increases your set point by 1 pound per day and your set point decreases between meals by 1 pound per day. This is a stable situation: Your set point will go up and

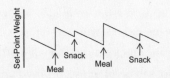

Figure 4. The effect of food on your set point.

down around the same value, day after day after day. January, February, March—your weight stays the same. On April 1 you change your diet so that your set point goes up only 0.8 pound per day. This is *not* a stable situation. Your set point goes down between meals more than it goes up at meals. The level around which your set point oscillates will gradually decrease—by 0.2 pound per day. Because this level is decreasing, you will lose weight. April, May, June, you lose weight. You will lose weight until you reach a weight at which your set point goes down only 0.8 pound per day between meals instead of 1 pound per day.

Idea 6. The stronger a food's flavor–calorie association, the more your set point will go up when you eat it.

The strength of the flavor-calorie association matters: Flavors strongly associated with calories raise your set point more than flavors weakly associated with calories. In "Applying the Theory to Everyday Foods," page 46, I will explain what makes a flavor-calorie association strong or weak.

You can get some sense of how strongly a flavor is associated with calories. A flavor not associated with calories tastes a bit flat and/or strange, or even unpleasant. As the flavor-calorie association becomes stronger, the flavor doesn't exactly change, but it becomes pleasant and familiar. You can experience this for yourself by drinking an unfamiliar tea. Add sugar to the tea (for calories). The first cup will taste mildly pleasant because of the sweetness of the sugar. If you have one cup of tea with sugar per day, subsequent cups will taste better and better as the flavor of the tea becomes associated with the calories in the sugar. If, on the other hand, you add a noncaloric sweetener (such as Splenda) to the tea, subsequent cups will *not* taste better and better. The tea's flavor will not become associated with calories because the drink has no calories.

You probably have several favorite foods that taste very good to you due to very strong flavor-calorie associations. These will always be foods that you have eaten many times. A chocolate-covered doughnut? A hot dog with a certain type of mustard? A glass of Scotch? If there are foods you crave, foods that bring great pleasure, foods you can't go a day without eating (if you are Pepsiholic, for instance), food you would drive thirty minutes for—those are examples. Eating these foods causes your set point to go up—more so than when you eat foods that aren't as familiar or flavorful.

At the low end of the strength-of-association scale are flavors not associated with calories. This is where every flavor begins. The very first time you taste any flavor, it has no association with calories. By the time you are old enough to read this book, however, almost everything you eat tastes at least somewhat familiar. The average person encounters completely unfamiliar flavors when being adventurous (going to an unusual ethnic restaurant, making a recipe with unusual ingredients or spice combinations) or when in a foreign country. I shop in many ethnic food stores, where I buy packaged foods with unfamiliar flavors—my version of armchair tourism. Eating unfamiliar foods does not raise your set point, so these foods offer a rare opportunity to fly under the radar of your body's weight-regulating system and eat without raising your set point.

Applying the Theory to Everyday Foods

How can we use this theory to figure out what to eat to lose weight? We need to figure out which foods when eaten many times have strong flavor-calorie associations and which have weak associations.

One hundred years of research on Pavlovian conditioning comes to our rescue here. This research has established two rules that have been found to apply to all examples of Pavlovian conditioning.

First, *the weaker the signal, the weaker the association.* If Pavlov used a bell that the dogs could barely hear, it would produce less salivation than a bell the dogs could hear clearly.

Applied to flavor-calorie learning, this means that *the weaker a food's flavor, the weaker its flavor-calorie association.* If you reduce the amount of flavor in your food, the flavor-calorie associations will become weaker. When I started eating large amounts of a relatively bland food (sushi) I did in fact lose weight. I later discovered that sugar water and extra-light olive oil—both of which have no flavor—worked even better.

Second, *the more delayed the outcome, the weaker the association.* In Pavlov's experiments, the bell was the signal and the food was the outcome. The food was given at the same time the bell was turned off. Had the food been given many minutes after the bell was turned off, the dogs would not have associated them at all.

Applied to flavor-calorie learning, this means *the slower a food is digested, the weaker its flavor-calorie association.* When a food is digested more slowly, the calories in that food are detected more slowly. Thus there is more of a gap between the signal (flavor) and the outcome (calories). I believe this is why low-carb and good-carb diets work: They replace foods that are digested quickly, such as bread, with foods that are digested slowly, such as vegetables. The foods that are digested more slowly have weaker flavor-calorie associations. They raise your set point less.

A Stone Age Grain Elevator

It's no great puzzle why our weight-regulation system works this way. It is a system designed to stock up on energy (calories)—that is, make us fatter—when food is plentiful and to reduce the amount of energy stored—make us thinner—when food is scarce. This is the way any sensible commodity storage system works. I stock up on paper towels when they are cheap and use what I have stored when they are expensive. Grain elevators store grain when it is cheap. The stored grain is sold when it is more expensive.

The system I've described uses the flavor of foods to determine whether food is plentiful or scarce. In Stone Age times of plenty, food tasted better. In the Stone Age, when food was plentiful the best-tasting foods—those with the strongest flavor-calorie associations—were more likely to be eaten than when food was scarce.

In the Stone Age, this system made us fat, or at least fatter, during "fat years," as protection against "lean years" to come. But nowadays, the lean years never come, and our once-precious fat does more harm than good.

Why Believe It?

No one believes a theory but the theorist, the saying goes. It's not entirely true. Two sorts of findings are especially persuasive. First, confirmation of a surprising prediction. A famous example is the return of Halley's Comet at the predicted time—very convincing evidence for the theory that comets orbit the sun. One surprising prediction of this weight-control theory that has been confirmed is that extra-light olive oil will cause weight loss. The usual idea has been that consuming fat causes weight gain. Second, repeated usefulness. When a theory is useful again and again, skepticism melts away. This theory led me to try a low-glycemic-index diet. That worked: I lost weight. It led me to eat lots of sushi. That worked. It led me to drink sugar water. That worked extremely well. It led me to drink extra-light olive oil. That worked extremely well too.

For more about the theory, see my paper "What makes food fattening? A Pavlovian theory of weight control" at www.sethroberts.net/articles/whatmakesfoodfattening.pdf.

～ Life Regained

STEPHEN Marsh, a fifty-year-old lawyer in Plano, Texas, learned about SLD in November 2005 from the *Freakonomics* blog. He weighed 245 pounds. He is five feet five inches tall so his BMI was 41 (morbid obesity). To get to his fourth-floor office, he had to take the elevator; the stairs were too hard. He had tried many diets; all had failed. With the Atkins Diet he had managed to get down to 225. The problem with Atkins was that it impaired his thinking. In measureable ways, his job performance suffered. Maybe there wasn't enough glucose in his blood.

Stephen started SLD drinking sugar water (SLD's early version). Within hours, he could tell that it was working. The sugar water was cumbersome, though, and he switched to ELOO. He varied between 3 and 4 tablespoons per day. By January 2006 he was down 25 pounds. As every SLD dieter says, it changed more than his weight. "Where I used to eat some donuts, be full and look around for more," he wrote, "now I look at the donuts and just don't feel like eating them. Instead of eating a slice of pizza and waiting until everyone leaves so I can finish the rest of the box, I lose interest in eating more."

As he lost weight, "emotions tied up with food or buried under food came to the surface," he says. "A lot of the emotion I had buried was positive emotion. Which was surprising. I didn't realize that I was as happy with my wife and kids as I was." Over the past twelve years, three of his children had died. "I started feeling grief instead of repressing it," he says.

He lost weight steadily (see below), although much of the time he felt he was not losing. What was the biggest difficulty? "Getting bored. There's no emotional tension in the diet. You take the olive oil, you eat less, you lose weight."

Now—after a year on SLD—he is close to his best weight. He has recovered all sorts of capabilities. He started doing judo again. In a recent tournament he managed to beat someone fifteen years younger. He can ski again. If he falls down while skiing, he can get up. He was able to participate in the recent renovation of his parents' house because he can carry things and use a jackhammer. He runs up the stairs to his office at least twice a day just to feel alive.

He feels as if he has regained his life.

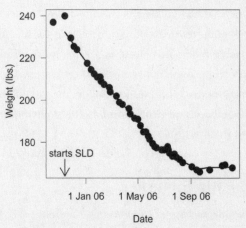

Figure 5. Stephen's weight over time.

4

HOW TO DO THE SHANGRI-LA DIET

Secretly, I suspected the answer to weight issues would be something ridiculously simple, but this is almost too much to hope for.
—*Starkville Daily News*

It appealed to my essential laziness.
—A BLOGGER'S REASON FOR TRYING THE SHANGRI-LA DIET

THE SHANGRI-LA diet is the most flexible weight-loss plan yet devised. No forbidden foods, no restricted foods, no calorie counting, no meal plans, no recipes, and, above all, no deprivation. No subtraction, just addition. Just follow the flexible basic framework and choose among the many possibilities it allows.

The Big Picture

The big picture of the Shangri-La diet is very simple. There are only four rules:

Rule 1. Take 200 to 500 calories of flavorless edible oil daily.

This corresponds to 2 to 4 tablespoons of oil per day because there are about 120 calories in a tablespoon of oil.

How much you should take, at least in the beginning, depends on how much you weigh. Consult the table on page 63 to choose a starting amount. After a few weeks or a month you may adjust the amount up or down to lose weight faster or slower. Don't try to lose more than two pounds per week. That's generally considered a healthy rate of weight loss. Most SLDers lose weight faster than that for a few weeks but then settle down to a long steady loss of about one pound per week. Because SLD is very easy and sustainable, this rate of loss is fine.

Rule 2. Take the oil at least an hour away from food and any flavors.

More precisely, you should take it *in the middle of a food-free, flavor-free two-hour window*. For example, if you expect to eat lunch from 12:30 to 1:30, take the oil before 11:30 a.m. or after 2:30 p.m.

The food-free and flavor-free window should have *no flavors of any kind*: no coffee, no tea, no toothpaste. Water is okay. Vitamins and pills that you swallow (rather than chew) are okay.

Other than the requirement to take the oil at least an hour before and at least an hour after any food or flavors, the time of day doesn't matter. The time of day doesn't matter because the oil is not a short-lasting appetite suppressant. Its effects last a long time.

You may eventually find you can take all your oil at one time. In the beginning, however, you will probably want to take the oil 1 tablespoon at a time—for example, 1 tablespoon between breakfast and lunch, another tablespoon between lunch and dinner, and a third after dinner. This is what most people do.

Rule 3. If the oil upsets your stomach, start small and work up.

To digest any food, we need certain enzymes. If a food is unfamiliar, we may not have enough of those enzymes at first, and the first few times we eat the new food it will sit in our stomach undigested, causing a stomachache. Whatever oil you choose for this diet, you may or may not be able to easily digest it the first time you drink it. If you have trouble—and about half of Shangri-La dieters do—don't worry: These problems almost always go away within a week. The oils I recommend have been consumed safely by millions of people for thousands of years; it is very likely that you too can consume them.

If you have any digestive trouble with the oil, you should start with a much smaller amount and gradually increase the amount. Start with 1 teaspoon per day and then, if you have no trouble with that, increase the daily dose by 1 teaspoon per day: The daily sequence of doses would be 1 teaspoon (e.g., on Monday), 2 teaspooons (on Tuesday), 3 teaspoons (on Wednesday), 4 teaspoons (on Thursday), and so on, until you reach the dose you want.

Rule 4. If you haven't lost weight after one month, increase your daily dose of oil by 1 tablespoon.

(But do not exceed 4 tablespoons per day.) People vary a lot, so it is impossible to predict exactly how much oil per day will work best for you. It is important for you to adjust the dose until you get good results. Judging by the SLD forums, the main cause of poor results seems to be not taking enough oil. If you are not losing weight and you don't want to increase the daily dose of oil, try the extra-credit methods in Chapter 6 ("Extra Credit: Eight More Ways to Lose Weight"). If you are not sure what to do, you can always post a question on the SLD forums (http://boards.shangriladiet.com).

What about the rest of what you eat? *Adding the oil is the only change to make in your diet.* You don't have to consciously eat less of anything or watch what you eat. You will be a lot less hungry, and you will find that you eat less and feel full faster. The overall result will be that you take in fewer calories and lose weight without making a deliberate effort to choose lower-calorie foods or eat less. A very nice feature of this diet is that it will help reduce or eliminate your cravings for junk foods. Most diets make life harder; this one makes life easier. See "In Shangri-La," pages 84–91, for many examples.

Which Oils?

For the oil to cause long-term weight loss, it must have little or no flavor (or must be consumed with your nose closed so that you don't detect its flavor—see p. 94). When I began using oil, for two years I used extra-light olive oil (the label may read *extra-light tasting* or *extra-light in taste*). Extra-light olive oil (ELOO) should not be confused with extra-virgin olive oil (EVOO, as Rachael Ray calls it). ELOO is less flavorful and lighter in color than EVOO, which is greenish. If an oil has a strong flavor, the flavor may become associated with calories. If this happens, it will eliminate the appetite-suppressant and weight-loss-causing effect.

Nowadays, I drink refined walnut oil and flaxseed oil because of their high omega-3 content

GOOD OILS

TYPE	COST PER 100 CALORIES	OTHER BENEFITS
Flaxseed	23 cents	Very high in omega-3
Refined Walnut	16 cents	High in omega-3
ELOO	15 cents	Part of Mediterranean diet

(see "Omega-3: Not Overrated," p. 58–61). Refined walnut oil is flavorless. Flaxseed oil is not flavorless, so I drink it nose-clipped (see p. 94) to eliminate the flavor.

In addition to omega-3 content, another important consideration in deciding what oil(s) to drink is the likelihood of unpleasant side effects. Of course, everyone is different so no one can predict in advance how you will react to any oil. But some oils cause less trouble than others. A poll on the SLD forums asked users of various oils to say whether there were unpleasant side effects. Here are the results (listing the oils from best to worst):

Oil	PERCENTAGE OF USERS HAVING TROUBLE
Walnut	8%
ELOO	25%
Grapeseed	33%
Canola	40%
Coconut	66%

Whichever oil you choose (particularly if it's high in omega-3), it will almost surely have positive side effects, such as better skin and softer hair. It is also likely to produce better sleep; as I mentioned in the Foreword, about three-quarters of SLDers report this. Among the many other positive side

Omega-3 is a type of fat. The name comes from the location of a double bond in the molecular structure of these fats: three carbons from the end (omega) of a chain of carbon atoms. Over the last sixty years, plenty of research has suggested that most people would benefit from more omega-3. SLD makes this easy: You are drinking oil anyway. Drink oil high in omega-3.

Early research about omega-3 involved heart disease. Why did Eskimos rarely die of heart disease, some scientists wondered, in spite of eating a high-fat diet (which was believed to cause heart disease)? The answer seemed to be that they ate a lot of seal fat, which is high in omega-3. During World War II, deaths from heart disease fell sharply in Norway and other Scandinavian countries. When the war ended, the heart-disease death rate returned to its previous level. The reason appeared to be that during the war, due to shortages, people in these countries ate more fish (high in omega-3) and less meat (low in omega-3) than usual.

Meat and fish differ in many ways, of course. Later research supported the idea that the difference in omega-3 content is what caused the difference in heart disease. One such study tracked the health of 22,000 doctors for almost twenty years. At the start of the study their blood was collected. By the end of the study, about 100 of them had died suddenly from heart failure. Their blood, which had been collected at the beginning of the study, was compared to the blood of a control group of about 200 similar healthy doctors. The most obvious difference between the groups—

clearer than lifestyle and genetic differences—was amount of omega-3: The dead doctors had less omega-3 in their blood than the healthy doctors. No other fat differed significantly between the two groups. The apparent effect of omega-3 was enormous. Doctors with omega-3 levels in the top 25 percent had a risk of sudden death 90 *percent less* than those in the bottom 25 percent. The benefit was not just huge, it was within reach. Because the "high" group—doctors with the highest omega-3 levels—was a large fraction (25 percent) of the subjects, we can be sure their diets were not extreme.

A well-known clinical trial called the Lyon Heart Diet Study showed the effect of adding omega-3 to the diet. It began in 1988 and ran for five years. It measured the effect of two different diets on people who had already had one heart attack. Half of the subjects were told to follow a low-fat diet recommended by the American Heart Association; the other half were told to follow a Mediterranean diet that included plenty of olive oil and canola oil. Among those who ate the Mediterranean diet, there were half as many deaths from all causes over the next four years as there were among those who ate the low-fat diet—a huge difference. Heart attack deaths in the Meditteranean group went down by two-thirds. The reduction in heart attacks became apparent within months of starting the diet.

Omega-3 also improves brain function, later research has implied. Because our brains are more than half fat, it makes sense that the wrong fats or too little fat may cause mental health problems. One connection is with mood disorders. Countries with low fish consumption, such as Israel, have much higher rates of bipolar disorder than countries with high fish consumption, such as Korea and Iceland. In some experiments in which patients with bipolar disorder or depression were given fish oil, these patients improved compared to patients not given fish oil. A survey of elderly Chicago adults found that those who ate more fish had less cognitive decline over time than those who ate less fish.

I became interested in omega-3 after it became clear that a side effect of SLD was better sleep. This suggested that fat could improve brain function. The only fat known to do so was omega-3; these improvements had been seen in people with mood disorders and the elderly. The SLD results suggested, quite plausibly, that omega-3 might also improve the brain function of the rest of us. This led me to increase my omega-3 intake. I found that my balance, my sleep, and perhaps my mood improved. (See my blog, at http://blog.sethroberts.net, for updates. I am studying these changes in detail.)

In our bodies, the omega-3 in plants is transformed into another type of omega-3 by an enzyme. The same enzyme also converts omega-6, a different polyunsaturated fat, into a different type of omega-6. There is "competition" at this enzyme between the two types of fat. When there is more omega-6, less omega-3 gets converted. This suggests that high levels of omega-6 can be harmful. There is evidence that this is true. The modern version of the Eskimo paradox is the Israeli paradox: Jewish Israelis have high levels of heart disease in spite of eating a diet low in saturated fat and high in polyunsaturated fat. The solution to the paradox appears to be that Jewish Israelis are eating the wrong polyunsaturated fat: They eat lots of omega-6, but little omega-3.

The practical implication of all this is that for SLD, you should use oils with low omega-6/omega-3 ratios. The best oils are:

	OMEGA-6:OMEGA-3 RATIO
Flaxseed	0.2:1
Canola	2:1
Refined Walnut	5:1

Among the worst oils are:

Corn	46:1
Sesame	137:1

Olive oil contains little omega-3. Fish is a good source of omega-3, but due to high price, mercury contamination, and overfishing, it is not clear that fish oil is a good oil for SLD. I get my omega-3 mainly from flaxseed oil, 1 to 2 tablespoons per day. To eliminate the flavor, I drink it nose-clipped (see p. 94).

The Queen of Fats (2006) by Susan Allport is a fascinating source of more information.

effects reported are fewer menstrual headaches, reduction of arthritis (which makes sense because omega-3 is an anti-inflammatory), better balance, and reduction of rosacea (a skin disease).

When choosing which oil to use, there are two things to remember. The first is that more omega-3 is better. This is not controversial; in the omega-3 sidebar (pages 58–61) I describe its best-known benefits.

The other thing to remember is that more omega-6 is bad—not quite proven to be dangerous but the evidence definitely points in that direction. Corn, soy, sunflower, and safflower oils are high in omega-6. In a 1971 study, men in the experimental group were given corn oil (high in omega-6). Their rate of cancer doubled over the next eight years compared to men in the control group, who continued to eat an average American diet. Before agriculture, there was much less omega-6 in our diet.

How Much?

Judging by the progress reports on the SLD forums, between 2 and 4 tablespoons per day of oil is usually an effective dose. I suggest you start with an amount that depends on your weight—see the table on page 63. If you are losing weight too slowly, you can increase the dose by 1 tablespoon per day (but do not go above 4 tablespoons per day). If you are losing weight too quickly, you can decrease the dose by 1 tablespoon per day. If (or when) you reach your target weight, you may want to reduce the dose so that you do not lose more weight.

To take much more than 500 calories (about 4 tablespoons of oil) per day of oil for a long period of time (months) is to venture into unknown territory. Consuming a great deal of any one food is usually a bad idea in terms of overall nutrition. Rather than increasing your intake above 500 calories of oil per day, I suggest supplementing the diet with one or more of the weight-loss methods explained in Chapter 6, "Extra Credit: Eight More Ways to Lose Weight."

The Two-Hour Window

The second rule is to take the oil at least one hour before or one hour after any foods or flavors—in other words, in the middle of at least a two-hour window during which you do not eat any food or flavored drinks. If you take the oil at a meal, it will simply act as added calories, strengthening the flavor-calorie associations of

WHAT A DIFFERENCE FLAVOR MAKES

Unflavored sugar water (see Extra Credit, page 93) and commercial soft drinks, such as Coke and Pepsi, differ by only a tiny amount, in the sense that the flavorings in Coke or Pepsi are a very small fraction of their weight (0.001 percent?). Yet this tiny difference in ingredients has a huge effect on how we respond to them. The difference emphasized in this book is that you can drink unflavored sugar water to lose weight; of course, you can't drink Coke or Pepsi to do so. Another interesting difference is that unflavored sugar water, unlike commercial soft drinks, never becomes addictive.

Dr. William Jacobs is a professor of psychiatry at the University of Florida's College of Medicine, where he specializes in addiction medicine and has directed the department's Overeating and Eating Disorders Clinic. He has never seen anyone addicted to unflavored sugar water, but he *has* seen hundreds of people addicted to commercial soft drinks, such as Coke, Pepsi, and Mountain Dew. A typical soft drink addict drinks two or three liters per day, said Jacobs. I believe that Coke, Pepsi, and the like can become addictive because they can produce very strong flavor-calorie associations. A food with a very strong flavor-calorie association tastes very good, which is why it is addictive; such food raises the set point a great deal, which is why soft-drink addicts end up at an overeating (obesity) clinic. Sugar water, without flavor, has no flavor-calorie association. Sweetness makes it pleasant to drink; but it never becomes addictive because without flavor there cannot be a very strong flavor-calorie association.

whatever you are eating. That's the opposite of what you want to do.

Many experiments with rats have found that adding sugar water to the diet causes weight gain. I believe this is because the sugar water is available at the same time as the rest of the food. The same may be true of taking oil with a meal. I spoke to a woman who lost weight while swallowing fish oil capsules between meals (for health reasons—she was doing the Shangri-La diet by accident) but gained weight when she began swallowing them at the same time as meals.

How far from meals should you drink the oil? I chose the value of one hour—in other words, the oil should be taken at least one hour away from meals—based on two sets of rat experiments. One set found that a flavor-calorie association was learned even when there was a thirty-minute gap between eating the flavor source and eating the calorie source. The other set found that a one-hour interval between flavor and calorie source was enough to prevent a flavor-calorie association from being learned.

Results tend to be better when people take the oil one hour after a meal rather than one hour before a meal. After taking the oil, you must wait an hour before eating something (water doesn't count). This is easier to do after a meal, when you're full, than before a meal, when you're probably hungry.

Your Real Food

The rest of what you eat, in addition to the oil, can be anything you want. However, an unhealthy diet is still an unhealthy diet. While you're losing weight, you'll be eating relatively small amounts of "real food"—that is, meals and snacks—because you simply won't be hungry enough to eat large portions. Make those small amounts as nutritious and healthy as possible. You may also want to take a multivitamin supplement as insurance to be sure you're getting adequate amounts of essential nutrients.

This finger-wagging tone doesn't do justice to how people actually feel about their food while on the Shangri-La diet. "I ate *pesto* yesterday (homemade) with lots of olive oil and nuts. . . . Pesto never would have been allowed on a conventional plan. Hooray!" (Homemade food is always a good idea.

See Method 4 in Chapter 6, "Extra Credit: Eight More Ways to Lose Weight," page 98.)

When you are losing weight, you will of course be eating less than usual because you will be a lot less hungry. My solution was to eat only one normal-sized meal per day. Sometimes lunch, sometimes dinner—it depended on who I was eating with. Some people who have done the diet have taken this approach, but most people have stuck with two or three small meals per day.

The Shangri-La diet works by itself, but if you are already on another diet plan feel free to continue it. The Shangri-La diet may help you stick with it (see "Other Diets at the Same Time," page 73).

What to Expect

Most people who try the Shangri-La diet notice changes within a few days, others almost always within a week. Based on the many blog postings, e-mails, and phone calls I have received from happy dieters, the first changes include:

- *Less hunger.* "Tried this diet for 2 days and I am not as hungry as I usually am." After just a few days: "It makes you feel so stuffed. Unbelievable."

- *Feel full sooner.* At meals, you will stop eating after less food. "This is the first time I have ever left food on a plate," "I'm able to feel full after eating about half of what I normally eat," and "I was a three slices guy; now one slice of pizza is enough" are typical comments. To eat the amounts you used to eat will become unpleasant. "I went to a buffet with friends last week and ate more than I meant to. . . . I felt really bloated afterward," wrote one Shangri-La dieter.

- *Think about food less.* One of my students tried the diet not because she wanted to lose weight but because she wanted to think about food less often. She carefully measured how often she thought about food before and during the diet. She was skeptical, she said, but it worked.

- *Fewer cravings.* A woman told me that for many years she had uncontrollable night eating. "I would wake up and crave something to eat, fall asleep, wake up and crave something to eat and so on. I would snack as much as three times during my sleeping time," she said. "I never slept through the night, never." The first night after she began the Shangri-La diet, it stopped. "I have gotten the best sleep in I can't tell you how long," she said.

- *Better food choices.* The Shangri-La diet is like power steering: It helps you do what you want to do. One dieter put it like this: "[Before the diet] I would say I'm not going to eat something sweet—and I would give in and feel bad about myself. . . . Now I eat an apple and I'm done. . . . I'm in control and I'm making the right decisions rather than the food is in control of me." Another person said: "It's true that 400 or 500 calories of oil/sugar consists of empty calories, but it has replaced, easily, about 1,000 calories of junk—soda, cookies, candy, chips. . . . Before, I could not resist the junk."

See "In Shangri-La," pages 84–91, for more examples of these changes.

How fast should you expect to lose weight? On a section of the SLD forums called "Post Your Tracking Data Here," more than 100 people on SLD have posted their weight at two or more dates. For both men and women, weight loss is faster during the first few weeks on the diet—men lose about 4 pounds per week, women lose about 3 pounds per week—than during later weeks. During Week 1 of SLD, weight loss varies with your weight. Heavier people, both men and women, lose more weight. After five weeks on SLD, both men and women lose about 1 pound per week. (For details, see http://boards.sethroberts.net/index.php?boards=15.0.)

In one of my experiments, one subject, a young man, did not start losing weight until seven weeks had passed. When the diet portion of the experiment began, he was slowly gaining weight, so it took longer for him to start losing weight than if his weight had been steady. A friend of mine doing the diet took the "you can eat anything" rule to mean that he could now eat fattening foods, such as ice cream, that he had previously avoided. He started eating much more of these foods at the same time he started the diet. He did not gain weight—as he would have pre–Shangri-La—but he didn't lose weight either. The problem was that the amounts of sugar water and oil he was taking weren't large enough to overcome the increase in fattening foods.

Almost everyone who does the diet has found that they need to adjust the dosage (sometimes up, sometimes down) to reach and stay at the weight they want.

Remember: *If you stop taking the oil, you will slowly regain the lost weight.* However, once you've reached your goal weight, you can skip days sometimes. If you find yourself regaining weight, just increase the dose on the days you do take it.

Possible Problems

Because the Shangri-La diet involves foods that are very common, it is almost always well tolerated. There is an important exception, however: people who have gallstones or who have had their gallbladder removed usually are advised to avoid fatty foods. If you have gallbladder trouble or no longer have one, be cautious with the oil. Start with very small amounts (one teaspoon per day) that you gradually increase. Cut back or stop if digestive upset occurs.

Other minor problems sometimes occur:

- *Difficulty drinking oil.* It may help to take very small sips at first. There is no need to drink the oil all at once. It may also help to add water (see "How to Drink Oil," page 66).

- *Headache.* This is common. It is probably caused by suddenly consuming less sugar or caffeine than usual in your meals and snacks— for example, less chocolate, less soda, less junk food. The headaches usually go away after a few days or a week.

- *Too little flavor.* You may find yourself desiring flavor—not calories, just taste. "I still have a lot of mouth-boredom/antsiness and want to just put something in there," wrote one dieter. As I mentioned in Chapter 2, "The Case of the Missing Appetite," I dealt with this by drinking tea, chewing gum, and eating supermarket samples.

Lessons From the Shangri-La Forums

The SLD forums, with more than 30,000 posts, report a vast range of experiences on the diet. I asked posters what they had learned from all that raw data. Here are some of the key things I've learned from their responses.

1. *People vary.* Some people experience appetite suppression on the diet within hours of taking their first dose of oil; for others, it can take days or even weeks.

2. *Don't be afraid to tweak.* The forums are full of stories describing how a person was having trouble with one way of doing things and then tried another way of doing things that worked much better. For example, a person might switch from ELOO to canola oil, or from canola oil to ELOO. Or might increase her dose of oil from 2 tablespoons per day to 3 tablespoons per day. It may take some tweaking to find what works best for you.

3. *Plateaus happen.* Even if SLD is working perfectly well for you, there will be plenty of weeks and possibly even months where you do not lose weight. This doesn't mean the diet has stopped working. Be patient.

Four years ago, for her term project, one of my students joined Weight Watchers. After a few weeks, she found it was hard to stay within the allotted points—to eat as little as the program requires. (Every food has a point value. You can eat no more than a certain number of points each day.) After she learned about my weight-loss ideas, however, she wondered if drinking sugar water would make things easier. She found that, indeed, 90 calories of sugar water per day made it much easier to stay within the limits, *counting* the sugar-water points. A friend of hers who joined at the same time but did not drink sugar water dropped out after three or four weeks. My student persisted and lost weight steadily. The combination of Weight Watchers and SLD probably worked better for her than either alone.

SLD has also been successfully combined with Dr. Barry Sears's Zone Diet. Terri Hill, of Boise, Idaho, was so successful with the Zone that in 2002 she was flown to New York and appeared on *20/20*. From 2002 to 2006, however, the stressors of life caused her to regain a lot of the lost weight. Part of the problem was birthday parties. (She has four grandchildren.) "You could eat a perfectly huge wonderfully balanced Zone meal," she says, "and then we'd have a piece of cake and ice cream. Before I'd be done with that piece I'd be hungry for another piece. Five hundred calories in the piece of cake. . . . I thought I was doomed to diabetes." She started SLD soon after she learned about it. Her appetite went way down; her craving for sweets went away. For her own birthday, "we bought a pie from Marie Callender's. I had a little bit. We threw the rest of it away. It was my favorite pie." When she did the Zone unaided, her failures worried her. "If you pop out of the Zone every week it messes with your mind, you're not at peace. Now I feel at peace. No matter what happens it will be okay. That feeling didn't come on until I was doing the olive oil."

In other words, SLD may help you follow other diets. It works the other way, too: Other diets may help with SLD. Someone posted on the SLD forums that she was not losing weight. "I don't even know if I'm getting appetite suppression or not because I eat out of habit . . . I don't know what hunger is." SLD works by reducing hunger. If you ignore how hungry you are, it may not work. Other posters advised her to try a structured eating plan such as Weight Watchers or TOPS. These plans would tell her how much to eat. She would no longer need to rely on figuring out if she was hungry.

⌁ End of a Nightmare

CATHERINE Johnson, coauthor of *Animals in Translation* and *Shadow Syndromes*, read about the Shangri-La diet in the *New York Times*, got a stomachache from too much ELOO, and forgot about it. She stumbled on the book nine months later and thought, *This is the answer to our life that I forgot.* Her nineteen-year-old son Jimmy is autistic. He cannot care for himself. Like many autistic children, he takes a drug that causes weight gain. After he started taking this drug, he began gaining about ten pounds per year. Late every evening he became hungry—so hungry and so agitated that his parents had to feed him what amounted to a whole meal. After four years of this, Jimmy weighed 220 pounds. His BMI was 32 (obese).

Catherine wanted Jimmy to lose weight, of course, but nothing had worked. Several times she and her husband had tried simply giving him less to eat. This failed. "He voraciously craved food," says Catherine. "The entire day, you'd be saying no. . . . All day long, he'd be screaming and biting. In the evening, there were hours of tantruming. It was hell, a constant nightmare." This was unbearable for more than a few weeks. And those hellish few weeks produced only a little weight loss. The only time Jimmy had managed to lose significant weight was when he attended summer camp. He took a long (1.3 mile) walk to camp and got exercise during camp. Unfortunately, this was unsustainable. "It was very labor-intensive," says Catherine. "I had to walk to camp and then walk home." That took too long. During sixteen weeks of camp, Jimmy lost six pounds. He gained all of it back when camp ended.

In July 2006, Catherine put Jimmy on the Shangri-La diet. Remembering her stomachache, she started at 1 tablespoon of ELOO per day. Later she increased it to 2 tablespoons per day. After several weeks, the effects were clear. In September, Catherine blogged: "Jimmy's nighttime bingeing is gone. We spent years of our lives dealing with a voraciously hungry, very autistic young man demanding food at 10 p.m. every night. It was exhausting, and now it's over. A miracle." He started losing weight, too (see Figure 6, page 77). By December 2006, he weighed less than 200 pounds, a loss of more than 20 pounds.

Catherine told her doctor, Dr. Erika Schwartz (www.drerika.com), a New York internist who specializes in treating hormone-related symptoms, about her son's success. Dr. Schwartz laughed. She had been giving some of her patients a weight-loss diet of her own devising, eerily close to SLD: 1 tablespoon of regular olive oil three times per day between meals. She had "prescribed" this to ten of her patients who had been struggling to lose weight. It helped all of them. "All ten of them lost weight fast. A few weeks later, they had lost 2 pounds, 4 pounds. They were very happy with the rate of loss. I immediately thought: placebo." But as the weight loss continued she began to think it was not a placebo effect. Her patients were healthy middle-aged women who weighed from 150 to 180 pounds. Dr. Schwartz's remarkable success rate suggests that SLD can help a large fraction of those who try it. There is no reason to think her ten patients were more likely than average to succeed with it; if anything, the opposite is true.

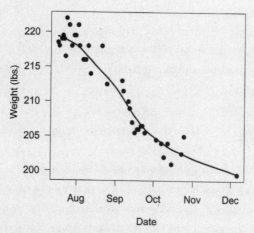

Figure 6. Jimmy's weight over time.

5

COMMON QUESTIONS

HERE ARE some of the most commonly asked questions about the Shangri-La diet, along with my answers.

Oil

[Q] *What kind of oil should I use?*

[A] For losing weight, ELOO (extra-light olive oil) is both cheap and widely available at large supermarkets, such as Safeway. If you would like to reap the benefits of oil that is high in omega-3 (see pages 58–61), then you should consider flaxseed oil (because of its flavor, you must drink it with your nose closed), canola oil, and refined walnut oil. If you have trouble with the first oil you try—if it doesn't cause appetite suppression or does cause long-lasting digestive problems—try another oil. See pages 56–58 for a discussion of differences between oils.

[**Q**] *Drinking oil is gross. How can I do it without gagging?*
[**A**] Adding it to a small glass of water and adding a bit of sugar will help. See page 66.

[**Q**] *How much oil should I take?*
[**A**] See pages 62–63 for a discussion of this question. The goal is to take enough oil to cause appetite suppression, but not so much that you don't get good nutrition from your ordinary food.

[**Q**] *Does the amount of oil change at any time during the diet?*
[**A**] If you think you are not getting enough appetite suppression, you should increase the amount of oil or use the extra-credit methods in Chapter 6.

[**Q**] *When during the day should I take my oil?*
[**A**] You can take it whenever you want, as long as you don't have any food or flavors (including toothpaste, beverages, and gum) for one hour before and after the oil. Many people find it convenient to take it first thing in the morning and last thing at night, so that half of the two-hour window occurs when they are asleep.

[**Q**] *Will I have to drink oil for the rest of my life?*
[**A**] Yes, unless you replace it with extra-credit

methods (Chapter 6). If you stop drinking the oil entirely you will slowly regain the weight you have lost. However, most people find that the oil has additional benefits (e.g., better skin, better sleep) and would be worth taking for those benefits alone. Think of the oil as something you take to stay healthy, like a vitamin supplement that just happens to help you lose weight.

The Two-Hour Window

[Q] *What is the two-hour window?*
[A] You take the oil in the middle of a two-hour period that is free from food and flavor sources such as coffee, tea, and toothpaste. Anything without a flavor, such as water and vitamins, is okay to consume during this period.

[Q] *Can I brush my teeth during the two-hour window?*
[A] No, unless you clip your nose to remove the flavor (see pages 94–96). The danger is that the toothpaste flavor will become associated with the calories of the oil.

[Q] *Can I drink things that have no calories during the two-hour window?*
[A] No, unless they have no flavor.

[Q] *I ate something during the two-hour window—is the diet ruined for me forever?*

[A] No—as someone said, "Tomorrow is another day." Just don't do it many times.

What to Do

[Q] *How can I survive Thanksgiving/Christmas/Holidays/Business Trips/Parties?*

[A] Think opportunity. On these occasions, it should be easier than usual to practice Extra-Credit Method 3, "Try new foods" (see pages 96–98). In general, don't worry about them. Because there are no forbidden foods on this diet, you can eat what everyone else eats and enjoy yourself. If SLD is working correctly, you will eat a lot less on these occasions than you used to. I remember a Thanksgiving years ago when I kept eating after everyone else at our long table had stopped. That doesn't happen anymore.

[Q] *What should I weigh?*

[A] There is scientific controversy about what weight is best in terms of life expectancy. The conventional recommendation has been that your body mass index (BMI), a measure of weight divided by height, should be between 18.5 and 25. Many Internet sites, such as www.nhlbisupport.com/bmi, will compute your BMI for you.

What to Expect

[Q] *How will I know if it is working?*

[A] You will begin to think about food less and,

without trying, find yourself going without food for longer than usual. Snacking will decrease or disappear. When you eat, you will feel full more quickly. When the effect is strongest, most SLDers lose interest in food most of the time.

[Q] *When does appetite suppression start?*
[A] A forum poll found that most people get appetite suppression within a day or so. For about one-tenth of those who answered, it took a few weeks or even a few months. The details are at http://boards.sethroberts.net/index.php?topic=3297.0.

[Q] *How long should I wait before deciding that it's not working?*
[A] At least one month, preferably two. A small fraction of people start to lose weight only after a month or two on the diet.

[Q] *Are there people for whom SLD doesn't work?*
[A] Yes, but I cannot yet predict who. I suspect that SLD works better the more junk food and packaged food you eat (although it works well for me and I eat almost no junk and packaged food). Also I guess that everyone's set point has a minimum value determined by their genes and life experience. Fattening food will raise your set point above your minimum, but nothing will cause your set point to go below your minimum. SLD can help you reduce your set point to your minimum, but not below that.

How It Works

[Q] *How can I lose weight by adding calories? That doesn't make sense.*

[A] You eat less later. The added calories of ELOO or other oil reduce how much you eat by more calories than you added. One hundred calories of ELOO, for example, may reduce your appetite so much that during the next day you eat 400 calories less (less snacking, smaller portions). The overall effect is that your calorie intake goes down. The ELOO has this effect because it lowers your appetite level, or set point.

General

[Q] *Does SLD help with emotional eating?*

[A] Yes. "My emotional eating has just about come to an end," one SLD forums poster wrote. Another poster made an interesting comment: "*Emotional eating* is a misleading term—we eat because we're hungry, and sometimes manage to keep ourselves from eating in spite of our hunger, but don't do that very well when we're unhappy. At least, that's been my experience." Someone else independently made a similar comment: "When I've gotten really good appetite suppression with SLD, it didn't matter how I was feeling—I just didn't have any interest in eating."

∽ In Shangri-La

But here, at Shangri-La, all was in deep calm.
—*Lost Horizon*

As THE introduction says, I decided to call this book *The Shangri-La Diet* because many people said the diet greatly reduced their struggles with food. Here are some examples from conversations, e-mails, and blog postings:

"Before this, I felt powerless over food. Diets never worked. It was just an addiction: I can't stop eating sweets, can't stop eating crappy food. Now I eat when I'm hungry."

"It's great to feel like I'm in control of things. Before my appetite was driving me; after eating I'd feel angry and guilty."

"I never eat the sweets at lunch anymore. Rarely at dinner. Now I'll look at something and think: If that's all they have and it's not that good, what's the point?"

"I can't believe the turn around [from] always wanting to eat to now eating at mealtimes and otherwise being content to pass it by. I even [blew off] an ice cream social. . . . This must be what freedom is all about. Free to eat, free to pass."

"[My] weight gain over the years had little to do with being hungry, but more [with] the reckless need to eat fattening foods such as bread and butter, dishes with cream sauces, cheese, ice cream, pastries and the like; it was more like an addiction to fat and carbohydrates. Following your recommendations helps control those urges, or perceived needs for "bad" things. . . . On Saturday I treated myself to light ice cream, and was perfectly content with 2 scoops (1 cup) for 240 calories."

"I saw the segment on *GMA* [Good Morning America] this morning. . . . I had gone to the gym at around six and had dinner around 7:30. I usually eat something else before I go to bed (popcorn, cheese) and I could feel the post dinner evening cravings setting in. I bit the bullet and swallowed a tablespoon of [canola] oil. Greasy but tasteless. Quite honestly, my cravings and desire to eat completely evaporated. 100%! And people, this never, ever happens to me."

"The most enormous difference I can see [since starting the diet a week ago] is that junk food—which used to sing its high-calorie, over-processed siren song to me loud and long, day in and day out—now holds only minimal appeal."

"I like cookies, and they are available at work. That's my problem. In these first two days, when I got the urge for some cookies, I drank the water.

That meant I drank a couple of tablespoons of fructose per day instead of eating a dozen cookies. . . . The net effect has been I've eaten much less sugar."

"I used to snack all day. In particular, chocolate. There's a steady supply around the office. But since I started this I've stopped eating the chocolate. . . . It simply doesn't occur to me to impulsively walk over and grab some, as I used to."

"My interest in chocolate has dropped dramatically—not completely, but dramatically. I generally keep a bag of little chocolate things around, like chocolate kisses. I'd go through a 2 lb. bag of Hershey's Nuggets in a couple of weeks. I'm going through them much less than half as fast."

"I just love the fact that I am not a slave of sugar anymore. I have such a sweet tooth and it is amazing for me to be able to say 'no thank you' to sweet temptations."

"Since I have been doing this, my between-meal cravings have all disappeared, and for the first time in my life I can look at something like popcorn, chocolate, potato chips, french fries, etc., and say 'I'm not hungry' and pass it up."

"It's just amazing how much my desire to snack has gone down. Don't have a whole lot of interest in it."

"I didn't realize to what extent my nighttime cravings were taking over. Now I come home and I just don't feel the need to snack."

"The best part of it is the snacking is cut out. Used to be a snacking frenzy at home after work while I'm cooking."

"I essentially cut all starches out of my diet permanently (I thought) because I just couldn't control myself around bread, cookies, bagels, etc. . . . Now, suddenly, I can eat a small amount of those things and not fall down the rabbit hole. Hallelujah."

"My weakness before the program was junky carbs—pretzels, breads, and the like. I noticed in the first week or two that my desire for carbs was significantly diminished."

"A few weeks ago I would have made a beeline [to the new Starbucks]. Now I'm just vaguely interested in perhaps going there to sit. . . . It is such a relief! I can still eat delicious things, but I'm definitely no longer entranced."

"This Thursday will make 1 full week since I've tried it. . . . I still eat 'regular food' but I have no cravings, and I end up eating a whole lot less as a result. . . . When I get home, I'm not famished and don't overeat."

"I started [six days ago]. . . . I was amazed at how quickly my appetite was under control. I say under control because I still ate but did not have constant cravings."

"I had a brownie at a conference last week. Took one bite and it was BITTER . . . . I wanted to spit it out of my mouth . . . I was so happy that I started chuckling to myself! I am a previous chocolate lover and if you told me that I would VOLUNTARILY turn down chocolate I would say that it was most likely because I was DEAD!"

"I have used the oil for a week now. It has changed my appetite. I was one of those that ate something salty and then had a need for something sweet and so on. It was like a never ending circle of cravings. I no longer have those needs to snack and cover the taste of the previous snack."

"Last week a neighbor dropped off a piece of chocolate cake and it actually went stale. I forgot it was there. Unheard of. . . . There is no willpower involved here. I still don't have any willpower. I'm just not hungry for those things."

THE SHANGRI-LA diet has reduced eating at night:

"[Before this diet, I] would sometimes wake up at midnight and eat 500–1,000 calories (sometimes more). . . . I have not eaten anything after dinner since I started six weeks ago, and not felt like I wanted or needed to."

"I became a night eater. I developed a habit—
even when I fell asleep, I would wake up and crave
something to eat, fall asleep, wake up and crave
something to eat and so on. I would snack as much
as 3 times during my sleeping time. . . . For the past
week between 9:00–10:00 p.m., I take a teaspoon of
EVOO. [Author's note: I suggest ELOO rather than
EVOO; EVOO may eventually stop working.]
Believe it or not, my hunger is gone during the night
and I have gotten the best sleep in I can't tell you
how long."

"I like to measure time by how long it takes to finish a box of Yodels. But I didn't even think about eating them. Normally I would eat them at night but I
didn't. I forgot about them."

"The diet works, it's easy, I eat whatever I feel
like, but I snack much much less, no late night nosh-
ing, and I don't miss it."

"After a week my wife could not believe that I
was not snacking at night (I always snack at night,
even when I am eating clean and watching what I
eat), but I simply was not hungry."

"No more late-night snacking, when I used to pop
a bunch of cookies or crackers or cheese things. No
chip cravings. It's the junk I've cut out."

THE SHANGRI-LA diet has allowed people to think
about food less:

"The constant thoughts I have about eating have subsided. One of the problems I have always had is that my brain is constantly thinking about food . . . what I'm eating, when I will eat, where I will eat and what I'm eating at the next meal, etc."

"I'm eating to live rather than the other way around."

"I'm so grateful for not thinking about food all the time."

"I have been able to stop thinking about food during times when I need to be working, cleaning, or playing."

THE DIET has made it easier to make good food choices:

"When I do decide to eat, I choose things that are good for me. No more junk food."

"I am able to make good decisions about how much I need to eat to keep my body going."

"[Before this diet] I would say I'm not going to eat something sweet—but then I would give in and feel bad about myself or I wouldn't and would be tortured by it. Now I eat an apple and I'm done. . . . I'm

in control and I'm making the right decisions rather than the food is in control of me."

SOME SHANGRI-LA dieters say it has given them more appreciation of food:

"I was seeing food as a negative thing because I kept gaining weight. Now I'm seeing it as the positive thing it is."

"When I eat sweets I enjoy it so much more—I savor it, because I'm not eating it all the time. I appreciate the richness of it."

6

EXTRA CREDIT: EIGHT MORE WAYS TO LOSE WEIGHT

FLAVORLESS OIL between meals should painlessly take you many pounds below your starting weight. For many people, flavorless oil alone is enough. A few daily spoonfuls of oil allows them to reach their target weight.

This isn't true for everyone, however. Some people don't want to drink oil or find that the largest dose of oil they can tolerate doesn't cause enough weight loss. Fortunately, the theory behind SLD (see Chapter 3, "A New Theory of Weight Control") suggests many other new ways to lose weight. I describe eight of them in this chapter. Each of them lowers your set point, the theory predicts; and, in practice, each seems to work at least some of the time. (People are too complex and varied for any theory to always be right.) I call these methods "extra credit" because most people will use them in addition to the oil. They are helpful but not always necessary.

All eight methods are based on the same basic principle: Foods with strong flavor-calorie associations are more fattening than foods with weak flavor-calorie associations; this is because they raise your set point more. And, for the same reason, foods with weak flavor-calorie associations are more fattening than foods with no flavor-calorie association.

Method 1: Drink sugar water.

The diet was first developed using sugar water. Chapter 2, "The Case of the Missing Appetite," describes how I found that drinking a few hundred calories of unflavored sugar water between meals caused great loss of appetite. I used this discovery to lose thirty pounds. My friends noticed, and the method spread. One person who tried it was a psychologist named Sarah, who used sugar water to go from a size eighteen to a size twelve. She started drinking sugar water in September; by Christmas she had lost twenty pounds. Taking a Christmas turkey out of the refrigerator, she realized, "I had lost a real burden"—the weight of a large turkey. She and her friends invented a weight-loss unit called the *turkey*: 1 turkey = 20 pounds. Eventually she lost two turkeys.

About one-fifth of those who post on the SLD forums use sugar water as part of their weight-loss regime. I find the side effects of oil so positive that I rarely drink unflavored sugar water anymore. If I want to lose weight, I drink more oil.

If you try SLD with sugar water, take 100 to 300 calories, or 2 to 6 tablespoons, of sugar dissolved in water. To prevent your blood glucose levels from becoming too high, you should drink the sugar water slowly, over thirty minutes or more. You can also use fructose, which looks the same as sucrose (table sugar) but is slightly sweeter and is digested much more slowly. (It has a much lower glycemic index.)

You should drink the sugar water in the middle of a two-hour window, separating it from all flavors by one hour before and after, just as you would with flavorless oil.

Method 2: Close your nose.

In June 2006, I got an e-mail from Gary Skaleski, a Wisconsin counselor. He suggested that closing your nose while you eat might make what you're eating as "flavorless" (as far as your set point is concerned) as flavorless oil. He remembered a high-school science demonstration in which an apple and an onion tasted the same if you held your nose while eating them. With a closed nose, salty, sweet, and the other tastes detected by your tongue are still present but the complex flavors determined by your nose are gone. Without being able to taste much flavor, perhaps 100 calories of any food will lower your set point and appetite as much as 100 calories of flavorless oil.

Gary and I, and eventually many other people, tested his idea. As far as we could tell, he was right: Eating something with your nose closed—usually by swimmer's nose clips ($3)—makes that food reduce your appetite much more than the same food eaten normally. If you eat a piece of pizza holding your nose, you will be much less hungry later than if you eat it normally. An SLD forum poll found that 85 percent of those who had tried "nose-clipping" (eating food with their nose closed) found it reduced their appetite. None said it increased their appetite.

This was quite a discovery. SLD was based on the idea that a few hundred calories of certain foods (such as flavorless oil) could cause a lot of weight loss. Use of flavorless oil to lose weight has limitations: (a) To get enough of other nutrients, you should not consume too much oil per day. Perhaps 400 to 500 oil calories per day is a good upper limit; (b) To drink flavorless oil requires planning. Flavorless oil is not everywhere. If you can replace flavorless oil with any food (eaten with your nose clipped), these limits vanish.

In practice, eating food with your nose held shut by nose clips takes a tiny bit of getting used to. You need to take small bites. There is also a big problem that never goes away: Your favorite food no longer tastes so good. To avoid this problem, people who eat food with their nose clipped restrict it to food they have no special feelings about, such as a banana. They also make smoothies with very healthy and nutritionally balanced components, such as flaxseed oil, fiber, fruit, and protein powder. Not having had prior experience with such a smoothie, they don't expect it to taste particularly good and are not disappointed when it doesn't.

Closing your nose is very easy and convenient and can make any food a weight-loss food. It does "look weird" and is slightly cumbersome, but this seems a small price to pay for the benefits. I love the side effects of oil and will never stop drinking it. But because omega-3-rich flaxseed oil isn't flavorless, I clip my nose when I drink it. After drinking the oil, with my nose still clipped, I take another drink of water to rinse out any lingering flavor before I take the clips off.

Method 3. Try new foods.

Foods with new flavors have no flavor-calorie association. Trying new foods can be as simple as buying new foods. In Paris, I lost weight because I drank new soft drinks. I like jams and jellies, but I avoid buying the same flavor twice. Rather than buy the same old frozen entrée, try a new one. Try a new flavor of soup. At a restaurant, order something new.

Restaurants with varying menus and daily specials make this easy. In *French Women Don't Get Fat*, Mireille Guiliano writes that "my business requires me to eat in restaurants about three hundred times a year." If these three hundred meals are at many different fancy restaurants whose menus change frequently, it is quite possible she rarely eats the same thing twice. Could this be why she has stayed slim? Dorie Greenspan, author of *Paris Sweets*, a cookbook about Paris pastries, told an interviewer that she's "always thought the [real] French Paradox is the way thin French women eat dessert three times a day [at cafés] and they're still thin." If they eat many different desserts at many different cafés—easy to do in Paris—this is no paradox.

The notion that novelty matters is new to the world of diets. At www.calorielab.com, an independent website about nutrition and weight loss, a blogger wrote, "I think we can say with a certain amount of confidence that things like the Starbucks 730-calorie Venti Caramel Chocolate Frappuccino with whipped cream fall outside the Shangri-La Diet." Well, no, not the *first* time you have it. Having it *once* is fine. This is not idle speculation. Recently I went to a special dinner celebrating the day on which James Joyce's novel *Ulysses* takes place (Bloomsday, June 16). Most of the dishes at the dinner were Irish, such as corned beef and cabbage. Dessert, though, was Italian: tiramisu, usually made with eggs, sugar, mascarpone, espresso, cocoa, and brandy or marsala. The Bloomsday version, however, used Baileys Irish Cream as the liquor. The portions were big; my piece probably had several hundred calories. But it tasted unfamiliar. I had had tiramisu many times. I had had Baileys Irish Cream many times. In spite of this, their combination was unfamiliar, which meant it qualified as new food. The next day I had remarkably little appetite and ate very little—due to the unusual tiramisu, I'm sure. The Baileys tiramisu was the opposite of fattening: It lowered my set point. This made me less hungry than usual the next day, so I ate less than usual.

Support for the idea that new-flavored foods cause weight loss can be found in *The Flavor Point Diet* by Dr. David Katz. The diet consists of eating only one flavor per meal without any calorie restriction. In practice, Flavor Point dieters eat almost nothing but new foods with unusual flavors. And it works, at least for a while: In twelve weeks, dieters lost an average of 17 pounds. The book has no data about what happens after that—when the new foods become familiar.

Method 4. Cook more.

The opposite of new food is familiar food, and the foods that can become most familiar are those that taste exactly the same each time—what I call *ditto foods*. These mass-produced foods come mostly from factories and chain restaurants. Because their flavors are so constant, when they are eaten repeatedly they can produce very strong flavor-calorie associations—much stronger than similar foods that vary in flavor, such as your homemade lasagna or meat loaf, which vary a bit each time you make them. (To increase the power of this method, I intentionally vary the flavors of my cooking.)

Ditto foods are the profit centers of the food industry. They include convenience food (such as frozen entrées, breakfast cereals, canned and frozen juices), ready-to-eat food, canned soup, junk food (such as soda, potato chips, and candy), fast food, and chain restaurant food. Almost any food sold in a package or made in a factory qualifies. It isn't just "bad" food; "good" food can be ditto food as well. "I've been having granola and soy milk for breakfast every day for months," wrote a woman who was trying my diet. "At first it made me extremely full until lunchtime. Now I'm hungry within a couple of hours." No doubt the granola was manufactured rather than homemade and tasted the same each time. And the soy milk tasted exactly the same each time. When she first started to eat the granola/soy milk combination, it was unfamiliar to her, and it acted like sugar water and flavorless oil: It lowered her set point. But with time, the flavors became associated with calories and became fattening. Chapter 7, "Changing the Rest of the World," explains why I believe the cause of today's obesity epidemic is an increase in the consumption of ditto foods—or, to put it another way, a decrease in home cooking.

Home cooks are neither machines nor fast-food restaurant employees following precise instructions with ingredients that are always the same. This is why a home-cooked dish usually varies from one rendition to the next far more than factory food or fast food. "The most successful dieters, we've found," observes Dr. Arthur Agatston in *The South Beach Diet*, "are the ones who try every recipe imaginable and take advantage of all the foods and ingredients permitted. . . . One patient invented a new soup made with every green vegetable he could find." The flavor of this soup surely varied a lot from one batch to the next. (And by trying new recipes, Dr. Agatston's most successful dieters were also following Method 3, "Try new foods.") Leftovers, unfortunately, are ditto food; so when you cook, make only enough for one meal.

Only foods that always taste the same become addictive. For example, a *New Yorker* article in 1995 by Susan Sheehan described an Iowa family that was living near poverty and seemingly headed toward bankruptcy. To save the price of a stamp, they paid bills in person. Yet the husband and wife both drank a lot of Pepsi every day, calling themselves "Pepsiholics." Almost every week, they ate dinner at McDonald's. "Going out to dinner is as necessary to me as paying water bills," said the husband. Other ditto foods produce similar behavior. As a high-school student, Jill Ciment wrote in her lovely memoir, *Half a Life*, she deeply wanted to save money to go to New York. She took on extra jobs, but couldn't manage to save anything. "I wasn't wanton with my money. . . . I just felt the dire need to reward myself for all my dogged hard work, to splurge on the extra candy bar, the jumbo Coke."

When In-N-Out Burger, a California chain, opened a new store in 1996, one of the first customers was a college student majoring in health education. "I was such a fan, I [had been] driving to Atascadero whenever I could convince somebody it was worth a three-hour drive," he told a reporter. "Now we have one here, and I'm in heaven."

Pepsi, McDonald's, candy bars, Coke, In-N-Out burgers—all ditto foods. Dr. William Jacobs, a professor of psychiatry at the University of Florida's College of Medicine, told me that the food addicts he has seen have usually been addicted to commercial soft drinks, ice cream, and certain fast foods, such as pizza and hamburgers—again, all ditto foods. He never saw anyone addicted to homemade hamburgers or homemade pizza. He also encountered people addicted to iced tea (with lots of sugar). The iced tea was both commercial and homemade; iced tea is so simple to make that even prepared at home it can taste exactly the same each time (especially if you use a mix). Addictive foods are addictive because they produce great pleasure. They do so because of a very strong flavor-calorie association. To build up a very strong flavor-calorie association, the flavor needs to be exactly the same each time you eat the food.

Method 5. Add random flavors.

An unusual way to vary the flavor of your food is to *add several randomly chosen flavors.* (A SLD forum member called this *crazy-spicing* and the name stuck.) One way to do this is to have many different flavor shakers, each with a different spice—basil, cumin, cinnamon, coriander, dill, garlic powder, ginger, mustard, paprika, pepper, nutmeg, oregano, and thyme—and season your food with a few of them, randomly selected. Even better is to use spice blends instead of spices. I have about twenty Penzeys Spices blends, such as Balti Seasoning, Jerk Pork Seasoning, and Beef Roast Seasoning. Each spice blend contains about ten spices. Adding a few randomly chosen spice blends to one's food is likely to create a completely unique flavor. Because the combination will be different every time, it will never become familiar. Dr. Alan Hirsch, a Chicago neurologist, did a study that suggests this will work. He gave participants flavorings to sprinkle on all of their food: two flavors each month for six months. Cheddar cheese (for savory foods) and cocoa (for sweet foods) were the first two, onion (savory) and spearmint (sweet) the next two, horseradish (savory) and banana (sweet) after that, and so on. Because the foods on which these flavorings were sprinkled already had flavor, this must have produced many novel flavor combinations. The novelty continued because the flavors changed every month. During the six-month experiment, the participants lost an average of thirty-four pounds. Those in the control group followed a traditional diet program and gained a small amount of weight.

You can take the first steps in this direction by simply adding a variety of seasonings to whatever ditto foods you eat. Instead of tasting exactly the same each time, these foods will now taste different each time, and as a result will be less fattening. In Chapter 7, on prevention, I discuss this approach at greater length. This method surprises many people, so let me be clear: I *am* saying that if you add cinnamon to your pizza it will make it less fattening, at least the first time you do it.

A problem with crazy-spicing regular food—such as pizza—is that it doesn't taste as good as expected, or as good as it usually tastes. A teenager would say the spices ruin it. As with nose-clipping regular food (eating it with your nose closed), you feel you have lost something. To avoid this problem, I rarely crazy-spice regular food. More often I make a very nutritious smoothie, with wheat germ, protein powder, yogurt, flaxseed oil, artificial sweetener (or sugar), and ice, all blended together. I add plenty of spices from randomly chosen spice blends. The result is pleasant (because of the texture, protein, sweetener, salt, and liquid) and unrecognizable. On a hot day or after a workout, they're great.

Method 6. Eat one food at a time.

My theory predicts that some foods are fattening because of what they combine; their ingredients eaten separately would not be fattening. I have eaten my share of pastrami sandwiches, for example. They taste very good to me because of the pastrami flavor. This is a sign that the pastrami flavor has become strongly associated with calories. Yet the average pastrami sandwich doesn't have many calories of pastrami. When I eat a pastrami sandwich, the pastrami and mustard produce a strong flavor signal; the bread, which has quickly digested calories, produces a large and quick calorie signal. The combination of the two produces a strong flavor-calorie association (see Chapter 3, "A New Theory of Weight Control," for explanation). Pastrami eaten alone would not do this: It doesn't produce a strong, fast calorie signal. The bread eaten alone would not do this: It doesn't have a strong flavor. Because pastrami alone and bread alone would produce weaker flavor-calorie associations, eating them separately (pastrami at 1 p.m., bread at 2 p.m.) would be less fattening—that is, would raise my set point less— than eating them together. (I don't actually do this; it is just a simple example to make the point.) With a pastrami sandwich, the meat and the bread happen to be two parts of the same dish. The general idea is that two dishes on one plate—roast beef and mashed potatoes, for instance—can act in the same way. By eating dishes at separate times, there is less of what I call *cross-conditioning*, and the flavor-calorie associations that develop are weaker.

This method of weight loss has been discovered by people not armed with my theory. It has an odd name: *food combining. Food separating* would be more descriptive, because it has rules such as "Do not eat fats with proteins" and "Do not consume starch and sugars together." The idea may have come to public attention in the bestselling book *Fit for Life* (1985) by Harvey and Marilyn Diamond. Suzanne Somers's popular diet books take this approach as well. I'm sure it works; it's just too hard to sustain. An Italian friend of mine went to a diet expert in Milan and was given a weight-loss plan that allowed only one type of food per meal. Monday lunch: vegetables. Monday dinner: protein. Tuesday lunch: fruit. And so on. It was very effective. Over five months, my friend lost about seventy pounds. Then he slowly gained it back, because the diet was too difficult. Four years later, he started the diet again and re-lost about seventy pounds. Then he re-fell off the wagon and slowly regained the lost weight. Quitting smoking is *much* easier than dieting, he says.

Less extreme versions of this approach are helpful, I believe. The French eat different dishes at different times during a meal. The vegetable dish is eaten separately from the meat dish, for example; the two courses might be separated by twenty minutes. This way of eating has the pleasant side effect of making meals easier to prepare, since there is no need to have several dishes ready at the same time.

Method 7. Eat foods that are digested slowly.

In Chapter 3, I discussed why food that is digested more slowly produces weaker flavor-calorie associations. In practice, until we can conveniently measure the calorie signals produced by fats and proteins, eating foods that are digested slowly means eating more foods with a low glycemic index and fewer foods with a high glycemic index (see box, below). There are several good books about how to do this, such as *The New Glucose Revolution* (2003), by Jennie Brand-Miller and colleagues. As I mentioned earlier, when I did this I lost six pounds. This was not earth-shattering, but it was so easy to continue to eat this way that I never regained the lost weight.

Low-carb and good-carb diets work moderately well. I believe this is because they replace carbohydrates that are digested quickly (high-glycemic-

THE GLYCEMIC INDEX

A food's glycemic index (GI) tells you how quickly its carbohydrates are digested. High GI = Fast digestion. Low GI = Slow digestion. For foods that are mostly carbohydrate, the GI is a good measure of the speed of digestion. The GI values of many foods can be found at www.mendosa.com /gilists.htm. A searchable database is at www.glycemic index.com.

HIGH GI FOODS	LOW GI FOODS
Most bread	Dried apricots
Dates	Grapefruit
Rice Krispies	Cherries
Instant mashed potatoes	Black beans
Baked potato	Lentils

index foods), such as bread, potatoes, and sweets, with foods that are digested more slowly, such as fats, proteins, and low-glycemic-index carbohydrates such as green vegetables. The slowly digested foods have weaker flavor-calorie associations than the quickly digested foods and thus raise your set point less.

Method 8. Eat foods with less flavor.

Weak flavors, like slowly digested foods, never become strongly associated with calories (see Chapter 3, page 46, for more on this). This makes foods with weak flavors—I'll call them *delicately flavored* foods—less fattening than other foods. It isn't easy to eat enough of these foods to lose significant amounts of weight. I tried to eat plain white fish—no seasonings at all—and gave up after one meal. Sushi was easier; I lost weight on my sushi diet. But it was hard to eat sushi day after day, not to mention expensive and unwise due to mercury in tuna. I believe that many meal-replacement drinks such as Slim-Fast are effective because they have weak flavors. They replace foods with stronger flavors. Much cheaper delicately flavored foods are widely available (see box, "A Few Delicately Flavored Foods," page 108).

While it is hard to eat food with little flavor, it is quite possible to eat food with *less* flavor. "I just leave off some salt, sweetener or sauce that I would usually use," one Shangri-La dieter wrote. "Next thing you know, I can't finish the plate of food. I can't live on bland, but once in a while it's a big help."

Behind the flavorless oil of Shangri-La Basic is the idea that the most potent weight-loss foods are those with *no* flavor. Timothy Beneke, an Oakland, California, writer, used this idea in a new way. In 1999, he weighed 280 pounds. His doctor told him he was nearly diabetic. Strongly motivated by this news, he used my early weight-loss methods (eat less-processed foods, low-glycemic-index foods, and weakly flavored foods) to go from 280 to 250 pounds. When I told him that I had lost weight drinking fructose water, he started drinking it too. By drinking 6 tablespoons of fructose per day, he lost about 50 pounds in nine months. At 200 pounds, however, he started regaining weight. I warned him that overshoot—more weight loss than can ultimately be sustained, as mentioned in Chapter 4, "How to Do the Shangri-La Diet"—was possible on the Shangri-La diet, but he interpreted the regain to mean that the sugar water had stopped working.

He stopped drinking it, and his weight went back up to 250 pounds.

After I told Tim about the good results I had with extra-light olive oil, he tried it. By drinking 3 tablespoons of ELOO a day, he lost weight steadily, reaching 210 pounds. At that point, his appetite returned and he had trouble staying at that weight. But he did not want to increase his daily amount of ELOO or resume the sugar water.

To provide a nutritious source of more flavorless calories, Tim inventively combined "liquefied fruits and vegetables, mixed with a powder made of brown rice, almond meal, flaxseed meal, dry non-fat milk, garbanzo powder, potato flour, and soy protein powder" (this description is from his web posting). He cooked the mixture until it was thick enough to make small clumps, then used a small spoon to form little pellets, which he swallowed with water as if they were pills. He simply ate some of this whenever he felt hungry, enough to make the hunger go away. He also ate normally (ordinary restaurant food, for instance) and continued to drink ELOO.

The mush worked, in the sense that Tim did not regain the weight he had already lost. "Doing 25% of my calories with mush and olive oil only kept me at 210 for 10 months," he wrote. But he didn't lose any more weight. Then, after ten months, he increased the mush to about 75 percent of his calories and found that he started losing weight again. Over five months, he went from 210 to 180 pounds, which he was pleased with. As of November 2006, he has stayed below 190 for more than a year. It isn't hard to get 30 to 40 percent of his calories from the tasteless mush, he has found. That amount is sustainable. "You get used to it. It becomes the norm," he says. More extreme than that, such as 50 percent tasteless calories, he has found he cannot sustain. A level of 30 to 40 percent puts his weight at about 190 pounds. This is quite an accomplishment because he eats very fattening food the rest of the time. When I interviewed him for this book, he told me the previous day had been typical of days when he is eating more than he would like. In addition to the tasteless mush, he had eaten two chocolate-chip cookies, a brownie, some Odwalla Green Juice, two or three chocolate-peppermint protein bars with milk, and potato chips. That was his food for the day.

Tim Beneke used my theory in a new way to sustainably lose *more* weight after first using it to lose eighty pounds. This is excellent support for the theory. Because the methods of this chapter are based on the theory, the more we can believe the theory, the more we can believe that the methods will work.

Beneke's method is extreme, but it is has produced great results. It is certainly far better—cheaper, safer, more widely available, and probably more sustainable—than another extreme solution, gastric bypass surgery.

If I Had Two Hundred Pounds to Lose . . .

If I had two hundred pounds to lose, the first thing I'd try, in addition to the oil, would be randomly flavoring all my foods, especially the ditto foods. I'd also cook as much as possible, replacing ditto food with homemade food and varying the spices. But the other methods have value too. I eat foods separately when possible; I have avoided high-glycemic-index foods for many years; I enjoy sushi now and then; and when a unique dessert comes my way, I eat it eagerly.

Overview: What Works Best

To get an idea of how these extra-credit methods compare to each other and to SLD (that is, using a flavorless oil, such as ELOO), I asked SLD forum readers to rate some of them on effectiveness and convenience. (I thank Brian Wansink, author of *Mindless Eating*, for suggesting this.)

The most popular SLD methods—rated highly effective *and* highly convenient—turned out to be (a) flavorless oil and (b) nose-clipped oil (that is, drinking oil with your nose held shut so that you don't smell it).

Moderately effective and convenient were four of the extra-credit methods, all with similar ratings: sugar water, nose-clipped smoothie, crazy-spiced regular food (regular food with random spices added), and crazy-spiced smoothie. The virtue of these last three methods, of course, is that they allow you to eat weight-reducing foods while getting excellent and balanced nutrition.

Nose-clipped regular food was rated as less convenient and effective than these other methods.

I didn't lobby for any particular outcome of this survey, but the results do a good job of describing my own SLD practices. Every day I drink flavorless oil (refined walnut) and nose-clipped oil (flaxseed). Now and then I add random spices to regular food. When I make hot chocolate from a mix, for example, I'll add small amounts of a spice blend or a few random spices to make the flavor less familiar. It still tastes good. On hot days I like crazy-spiced smoothies, to which I often add granola for texture. Sweet, creamy, cool, thirst-quenching, crunchy, spicy: They can be delicious.

⤳ The Blogosphere Tries It

AFTER A *Freakonomics* column about the Shangri-La diet appeared in *The New York Times Magazine* (September 11, 2005), Stephen Dubner and Steven Levitt, the authors of the column, kindly invited me to guest-blog at www.freakonomics.com. Something unexpected happened: People started posting their experience with the diet. The very first report was negative:

> "I tried a tablespoon of extra-virgin olive oil yesterday and of canola oil today. . . . Neither one did anything for my hunger, I ate just as much as usual at my subsequent meals."

THEY SOON became overwhelmingly positive:

> "I don't need to lose weight but I must say this sugar water stuff works like magic for me."

> "Whoa. Close to zero appetite. . . . Ridiculously easy. And cheap. And effective. What hath God wrought?"

> "I've lost 6 lbs. in 5 days, despite eating better than I have in years. . . . For me, the debate is over. I've never been able to lose weight so effectively—not even

on a raw foods diet or when athletically swimming four hours a week."

"When I started this, I weighed 226. I now weigh 220.5. Not bad for 9 days. . . . My diet is as varied and as nutritious as ever, perhaps more so."

"I've lost about 3 pounds in ten days. Not earth shattering, but slow and steady is good I think."

"Your conclusions on fructose sugar are right on the money. I've got 20 lbs. of weight loss so far to prove it."

THERE WERE a few failures too:

"I tried fructose water for 3–4 days and GAINED THREE POUNDS!!! 45–60 minutes after drinking the sugar water I WAS RAVENOUS!!!"

"I've tried the regime for about two weeks now with no results. I've been drinking 250 calories of fructose dissolved in a liter of water. . . . I haven't gained weight, but I haven't lost any either."

BILL Q. wrote at www.freakonomics.com: "I've been on the diet for three days. I've lost seven pounds. I've not had a moment of hunger, nor have I experienced any odd cravings." He added that he would post later results at his blog "assuming the program is a success." No later results appeared, suggesting that the program failed.

After my freakonomics.com stint, Ann Hendricks set up Annie's Shangri-La Diet Blog (http://annhendricksshangrila.blogspot.com) so that people trying the diet could share their experiences. As of January 2006, there were about two hundred posts. They told the stories of nine people:

DE BENCI, starting at 185 pounds, lost 8 pounds over eight weeks, making only changes "that I feel I can stick with in the long term." He successfully used honey water instead of sugar water.

EMILY started at 276 pounds. Over seven weeks, she lost fourteen pounds. "It is very interesting to feel like I might have some measure of control over my weight. Previously, I have tried the standard diet and exercise method and have felt hungry, deprived, and frustrated."

JULIE had little luck. She lost a few pounds at first but then stopped losing. Eventually, "I stopped drinking my sugar water because I didn't think it was working for me. I gained back the weight I lost."

LEFTBLANC started at 226 pounds. Over eleven weeks, he lost 25 pounds. (See page 121 for more about his experience.)

MASA'IL (Hendricks herself). Starting at 192 pounds, she was down to 176 pounds—eighteen pounds lost in eleven weeks. The diet, in her experience, is "definitely irreplaceable so far: Nothing [else] has helped me as much."

MICHELLE started at 170 pounds. Over five weeks, she lost fourteen pounds. "I'm definitely making better choices when I do eat," she wrote. "Food is still very appealing to me, but I'm drawn to good food and proper portions. It's not effortless or even particularly easy, but it does seem possible." She began to feel skeptical, yet still hopeful, after she skipped her Shangri-La routine for a few days and her hunger returned. However, getting back on the diet did not immediately curb her appetite.

MOLLY. After two weeks, she wrote: "Jeez, this diet makes me so hopeful it's almost scary. I've fought my weight my whole life, and the idea that I might actually be able to reach my ideal weight and stay there is . . . the word *miraculous* keeps coming to mind. No dangerous drugs? No diet restrictions like no carbs, or no fats? No grinding hunger? And I can eat and enjoy pleasurable foods? It boggles the mind." After three weeks, she had lost six pounds, and wrote: "So much of what I previously thought about weight loss, diet and nutrition seems useless in light of my experience on this diet." The most recent summary I have of her experience is: "I lost 12 pounds [in eight weeks, starting at 155], then went on vacation for 2 weeks and (stupidly) gained back 6, of which I have now re-lost 3 (in 4 days)." The diet "is a very useful tool for controlling eating while trying to lose weight," she wrote. "And I'm very grateful for that."

SARAH's first post said that she had been "doing the diet for almost 2 weeks. It is working like a dream. . . . I feel great, I've got energy to work out for more than an hour, and I am really, really excited that this is working so easily. I have lost about 4 lbs. and that is big since I am trying to lose the last 15 of a 100-lb. weight loss and before now, it just would not budge." She lost weight steadily. Three weeks later, in her last post, she wrote, "I have nothing to report except consistent, slightly boring weight loss with not a lot of effort—which of course is huge and unprecedented for me."

SFC started at 184 and over three months steadily lost eighteen pounds. "This has been nearly effortless," he wrote. "My food cravings are down, my appetite is down, and I very, very seldom eat more than 2,000 calories a day, which before I started was more like my minimum calorie consumption." After he e-mailed me, I spoke to him by phone. He said he lost the weight without any exercise—a deliberate choice. During the first eight weeks, he had drunk up to 500 calories per day of fructose water; then he switched to mostly extra-light olive oil. The oil worked as well as the fructose water.

THE RESULTS were so consistently positive that Hendricks eventually asked people to post other outcomes:

"Getting the real range of experiences posted would definitely be the best way to really explore this thing. . . . Any failures or 'less-than-spectacular successes'?"

AFTER THIS, two people posted:

ROBERT F. wrote that he had "tried the diet over the past two months with only minimal success." (I believe his dose of sugar water was not large enough to overcome his "resumption of eating carbs.")

AGNOSTIC wrote, "I lost 5 pounds in 3 weeks [but] I haven't lost any [more] weight for a month now."

SOON AFTER the *Freakonomics* column, www.calorielab.com, an independent website about nutrition and weight, posted a long article about the diet. Bottom line: "If you had to cook up the ultimate stereotype of a wacky fad diet for use in a comedic novel or film, the Shangri-La Diet would fill the bill." However, "we're not necessarily saying it won't work." The article discussed the ideas behind it, adding "we suspect he cooked it [the theory behind the diet] up as an afterthought to justify his development of a weight-loss program while being employed as a psychology professor."

(Actually, the theory came first.) Then the success stories, posted as comments to the CalorieLab report, began:

"I am two weeks into the oil diet. . . . I have lost three pounds. Was 168. lbs, 5'11". . . . Appetite much suppressed. Not much determination required to take small helpings. Eating is oddly optional after a very small meal."

CALORIELAB noted that people eat for reasons other than hunger, thus "a system like Roberts's that supposedly suppresses actual gimme-energy hunger is not going to work long term, once the initial excitement of trying a new diet wears off." The successful dieter replied:

"Separating, through this diet, gimme-energy hunger from the other motivations to eat has been instructive. The other motivations are much clearer. . . . They are easier to control because the gimme-energy hunger is suppressed."

THE SUCCESS stories continued:

"I am 54, 5'8" post-menopausal at 146 lbs. I have been on this program for 10 days and have lost 4 pounds. . . . I am delighted with the current cut in appetite."

"I have been using the 'Shangri-la' diet now for almost a month, and it works beautifully. It has re-

moved my cravings and registers a full stomach whenever I eat."

CALORIELAB replied: "Remember: The whole diet may be nonsense and not work." But then:

> "Have been doing this for 3 weeks. . . . Have lost 11 pounds and it's been easy."

> "I just have to say it works. I tried it for 2 weeks. . . . I have lost my extra fat around the waist I had after having 3 kids."

A *Good Morning America* segment about the diet on November 14 produced a burst of questions, which CalorieLab patiently answered, adding, "We think this is just a crazy fad diet." The mini–success stories continued:

> "I've been following your Shangri La guidelines now for 3 days. . . . It does appear to work as an appetite suppressant."

> "My family doctor recommended that I try this diet as a safe alternative to prescription weight-loss medication. . . . Olive oil helps increase HDL (good) cholesterol. So even if it doesn't help you lose weight, it looks like it may have a few other advantages. I have used the oil for a week now. It has changed my appetite."

LEFTBLANC, who had posted extensively at Annie's Shangri-La Diet Blog, told www.calorielab.com readers that "I started this diet on 9/12 . . . I am 5'11", and weighed 226 pounds. I now weigh 205 pounds" (November 23). CalorieLab replied, "Have you tried a more traditional calorie counting diet and not been able to stick to it? . . . I suspect that water or hot water in itself has an appetite suppressing effect simply by filling up your stomach," and went on to suggest a more traditional weight-loss plan ("avoid calorie-dense fast food, restaurant food, and packaged food"). Here is a bit of Leftblanc's long response:

"Why would I avoid restaurant food? I live in New York City, home to some of the greatest restaurants in the world. . . . This diet allows me to lose weight with a minimum of effort (and hunger). It's so much easier than counting calories. It's not like I didn't know a jelly doughnut had a lot of calories [during the seven years I weighed 226]; I ate it anyway."

STEPHEN M. joined the discussion:

"I can't say enough about the dramatic switch in the way I feel about food. I'm learning to think normally and act normally."

STARTING AT 240 pounds, he reported losing 15 pounds after 5 weeks. Yet another success:

"I'm a 52-year-old woman, 5 feet tall. I've been on the Shangri-La diet since September 17, 2005, and have gone from 163.50 pounds that day to 144.125 pounds today." [November 28. She lost nineteen pounds in eleven weeks.]

ALTHOUGH most comments have been positive, not all of them have been. On December 23, Imtiaz wrote:

"I have been trying the oil for about 8 days now and have not noticed any change in my appetite."

The blogosphere, so far, likes the diet—a lot. Maybe people are more likely to report success than failure, but this is a very promising beginning. At the SLD Forums (http://boards.shangriladiet .com) you can find hundreds of similar stories, including long-term results.

7

CHANGING THE REST OF THE WORLD

I didn't know any English at all when we came to the States. I knew hello, thank you, good-bye, *and for some obscure reason I knew the word* gluttony.

–KHALED HOSSEINI,
AUTHOR OF *The Kite Runner*

In the year 2001 so many physical problems will have been surmounted that . . . a woman will have a strong supple and splendid body all her life.

–1967 MEMO FROM DIANA VREELAND
(*Vogue* EDITOR IN CHIEF)

WHEN YOU understand what causes a problem, it becomes much easier to fix it. The reverse is true too: If you can efficiently fix a problem, it suggests you understand what caused it. Flavorless oils will not only help people lose weight, they will help teach what causes obesity and how to prevent it.

This chapter is about prevention. Previous chapters have described solutions that are fairly easy and clear and that can begin tomorrow. This one is about solutions that require more effort, patience, persuasion, and thought.

A basic principle of problem solving is that the

forces we can create, that we completely control, that we can turn on and off at will, are usually much weaker than preexisting forces we cannot turn on or off but merely point in a new direction. When a problem needs to be solved, I can do something whose sole purpose is to solve it (the direct approach) or I can modify what I was going to do anyway for other reasons (the preexisting force approach). If I need toothpaste, for example, I can take a trip to the store (direct) or I can wait until my other trips take me near a store (preexisting force). To get more exercise, I can go to a gym (direct) or I can start walking to work instead of riding the bus (preexisting force: I am already going to work). This chapter is about how two powerful preexisting forces—teachers and the food industry—can help prevent obesity in light of the ideas of this book.

What Caused the Obesity Epidemic?

To do something about the obesity epidemic, it helps to know what caused it. In 1962, a large survey found that 13 percent of adult Americans were obese. In 1980, that percentage was 14 percent—essentially the same. By 1993, however, it was 22 percent and by 2000, 30 percent—a huge increase. Something very fattening began between 1980 and 1993.

What was it? Too little exercise, high-fat foods, soft drinks, and too-large portions are often blamed, but so are many other things. In *Food Fight* (2004), Kelly Brownell and Katherine Horgen point to several causes: television, video games, personal computers, eating away from home, snacking, and "the glorification of overeating." However, the evidence for most of these causes has been far from persuasive.

The sharp rise in obesity after 1980 is unlikely to be due to lack of exercise. First, there was no sharp drop in exercise after 1980. Time spent watching TV increased by 45 percent from 1965 to 1975, yet obesity increased little over that time; from 1975 to 1995, when obesity shot up, TV watching increased only a little. Second, if lack of exercise were a big cause of obesity, then getting more exercise should be a good way to lose weight. It is not. Unless you are completely sedentary to begin with, it is difficult to lose much weight through exercise alone. Oprah Winfrey provided unwitting proof of this when she started running half marathons. That's how fit she had had to become—to put it another way, how much exercise she had needed to do—in order to lose the weight she wanted to lose. In the 1950s, Americans were much thinner than now, but not because they were more active; if anything, they were less active. The President's Council on Physical Fitness was created in 1956 to address an alarming lack of fitness.

The obesity epidemic is unlikely to be due to a high-fat diet. In the 1950s, Americans were not eating low-fat diets, yet they were much thinner. Another reason to doubt that high-fat food is a common cause of obesity is that, when studied experimentally, low-fat diets produce little weight loss. After a year, most people have lost only a few pounds.

The obesity epidemic is unlikely to be due to larger portions. From 1976 to 1996, calorie intake at breakfast, lunch, and dinner increased little, if at all; rather, there was a big increase in snacking. Restaurant portions have grown over the years, but I believe this is an effect of obesity rather than a cause of it. Restaurant portions did not physically grow during the three months I lost thirty-five pounds, but they came to appear huge—far more than I wanted to eat. Even after I stopped losing weight, they still appeared too large. My metabolism had slowed down. Likewise, when people gain weight their metabolism speeds up. They eat more and require larger portions to feel full.

So what *did* cause the obesity epidemic? The theory behind the Shangri-La diet (see Chapter 3, "A New Theory of Weight Control") is very clear. The most fattening foods, it says, are those that have all four of the following properties:

- A strong flavor.

- Quickly detected calories.

- Have been eaten many times.

- Have exactly the same flavor each time.

Might the consumption of such foods have greatly increased after 1980?

Junk food and fast food have these four properties; in fact, they have been engineered to have them. The table on page 128 gives some examples. Has consumption of these foods grown dramatically since 1980? The answer is yes. The economists Inas Rashad, at Georgia State University, and Michael Grossman, at the City University of New York Graduate Center, considered several possible causes for the obesity epidemic. "As much as two-thirds of the increase in adult obesity since 1980," they wrote, "can be explained by the rapid growth in the per capita number of fast-food restaurants and full-service restaurants, especially the former." Between 1960 and 1980, the per capita number of such restaurants grew slowly. After 1980, the number grew quickly. Figure 7, page 129, shows how closely the rise in obesity mirrored the rise in restaurants. From 1978 to 1996, calories eaten in sit-down restaurants doubled; calories eaten in fast-food restaurants tripled.

It's not just junk food and fast food. What I call ditto foods (foods that taste exactly the same each time) usually have these four properties as well. Ditto foods are not only found in restaurants and vending machines. You also eat them at home whenever you eat processed foods that need little or no preparation: Breakfast cereals, microwaveable entrées, frozen pizza, crackers, orange juice from

THE FOUR PROPERTIES THAT MAKE FAST FOOD AND JUNK FOOD SO FATTENING

FOOD	STRONG FLAVOR FROM . . .	QUICKLY DETECTED CALORIES FROM . . .	UNIFORM FLAVOR FROM . . .	EATEN MANY TIMES BECAUSE . . .
Soft drink (Coke, Pepsi)	Secret ingredients	Glucose in high-fructose corn syrup	Mass production	Sold everywhere
Hamburger (McDonald's, Wendy's)	Ketchup, mustard, pickles, onions, secret sauce	Hamburger bun, French fries eaten at the same time	Standardized preparation, mass-produced ingredients	Sold everywhere
Pizza (Pizza Hut, Domino's)	Tomato sauce, toppings	White flour in crust	Standardized preparation, mass-produced ingredients	Sold everywhere
Doughnut (Krispy Kreme, Dunkin' Donuts)	Fillings, toppings	Sucrose, white flour	Mass production	Sold everywhere
Chocolate bar (Snickers, Mars)	Chocolate, flavorings	Sucrose	Mass production	Sold everywhere

a carton, and cookies are just a few examples. The general name for these is *convenience foods*. They are made in factories. They are supposed to taste exactly the same each time. In a 2003 paper, Harvard economists David Cutler, Edward Glaeser, and Jesse Shapiro, who knew nothing about my

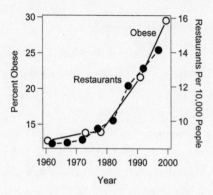

Figure 7. The growth of obesity in the United States from 1960 to 2000 closely parallels the growth in the number of restaurants.

ideas, argued that the obesity epidemic was due to a great increase in the consumption of convenience foods (or, to put it another way, a great decrease in food preparation time) from 1978 to 1996. They had many types of evidence for this conclusion. For example, they found that the more reduction in food preparation time for various demographic categories (married women, single women, married men, single men) the greater the weight increase of persons in that category. Married women had the largest decrease in time spent preparing food, and gained the most weight.

Taken together, these ideas and facts give us good reason to think that the obesity epidemic is caused by eating too many foods with strong flavor-calorie associations. If this is correct, what should we do?

What Teachers Can Do

Obesity prevention naturally begins with children. After taking a tour of the Edible Schoolyard, a school garden in Berkeley, California, I asked an eighth-grader what she thought of it. She liked it, she said, because it had made her a better cook. "It's made me eat foods I didn't eat before. My mom's a good cook, though." Well, why didn't her mom's cooking have that effect? Because she refused to eat anything her mom made.

If a child's culinary mind is open only away from home, how can we take advantage of that? Dr. Antonia Demas, a food educator who founded the Food Studies Institute in upstate New York, may know better than anyone else how schools can persuade students to eat new foods.

In the late 1960s, Demas began to volunteer at a local Head Start center so that her infant son would be around older children. The food served there appalled her and she concentrated her volunteer efforts on improving it. Part of the problem was how to make the kids eat better foods. The solution, she noticed, was that the kids would eat anything they had helped make. So she taught them how to cook. Later, she volunteered in a second-grade classroom and continued to teach about food, connecting it with the teacher's lesson plan in creative and interesting ways. When the lesson topic was Native Americans, for example, she helped the students make traditional Iroquois corn soup, and compared flint corn to sweet corn. When the topic was archaeology, she told the students about the Bog People, ancient bodies discovered in the peat bogs of northern Europe. Because peat preserves soft tissues, researchers were able to determine their last meals, which were usually assortments of whole grains. So her students cooked a porridge of whole grains. Every two weeks Demas did another unit. "It stretched me in very creative ways," she said.

In the early 1990s, Demas decided to get a Ph.D. at nearby Cornell to document her curriculum development and make it available to other teachers. She conducted her dissertation research, a simple experiment, at a local elementary school. Half of the school's teachers agreed to let her teach units in their classes. They were the treatment group. The remaining twelve classes, taught by other teachers, did not receive Demas's curriculum. They were the control group.

She taught sixteen different lessons, with sixteen different foods, in each of the twelve treatment classes. For a lesson on India, the students made curry, a mixture of spices, sweet potatoes, carrots, and lots of other vegetables, with brown rice on the side. For a lesson on North Africa, the food was a stew of chickpeas, beans, tomatoes, zucchini, and other vegetables, with whole wheat couscous. From the point of view of obesity prevention all of these foods were excellent. Their flavors were unfamiliar, they contained no source of quickly detected calories, they were homemade and complex, so the flavor would vary quite a bit each time they were made, and they were not widely available.

After she had given a particular lesson in all twelve treatment classrooms, the food cooked at that lesson was served as a side dish for lunch in the cafeteria. It was not optional: It was put on every child's tray. After lunch, each side-dish container was weighed to determine how much of the food had been eaten.

The main result was very clear. Children in the treatment classes usually ate most or all of the side dish. Children in the control classes almost always ate none of it.

The lessons had other effects. As the year progressed, children in the treatment classes ate more and more of the lesson foods at lunchtime. They became more and more used to trying the new foods they had cooked. From conversations that Demas overheard, she learned that it had become cool to eat as many different foods as possible and to eat unusual foods.

The effects went beyond the school cafeteria. The kids took the recipes home and made them for their families. They told their parents about the virtues of the ingredients. They got excited about cooking. Demas ran into parents at the supermarket. "I can't believe it," the parent would say. "My kid wants to eat this food, wants me to buy ingredients so she can prepare it." They would never have believed that their kids would want to eat any of this food, much less want to prepare it.

After receiving her Ph.D. in 1995, Demas helped start similar teaching programs in Santa Fe, New Mexico, and Rochester, New York. Today, her work is used in more than four hundred schools. In Santa Fe, the program, called Cooking with Kids, has grown from two schools to ten schools, with about four thousand students participating. Demas continues her research. In South Bend, Indiana, she recently completed a study in which she was able to learn what the parents of children in her program bought at the supermarket. Purchases of the more unusual foods, such as collard greens, escarole, and bulgur wheat, went way up, and the increases lasted at least six months after the program ended. Three-quarters of the children in her program lost weight. It's an excellent start.

Another way to improve what children eat is suggested by a story in *Totto-Chan* (1981), a memoir by Tetsuko Kuroyanagi, a TV star in Japan, of her elementary-school days. Kuroyanagi attended a small private school in Tokyo during World War II. On Sports Day, a Japanese national holiday, schools everywhere have athletic competitions. One of many wonderful and special things about Kuroyanagi's school was that the Sports Day prizes were vegetables: "First Prize might be a giant radish; Second Prize, two burdock roots; Third Prize, a bundle of spinach," wrote Kuroyanagi. The children grumbled about these prizes, so the headmaster spoke to them. "Get your mothers to cook them for dinner tonight. They're vegetables you earned yourselves. You have provided food for your families by your own efforts. How's that? I bet it tastes good!" Kuroyanagi added, "He was right." It's not just an interesting idea; it's an interesting idea that worked.

What the Food Industry Can Do

In the battle against obesity, big food companies are not the enemy, as many public health advocates seem to think. This belief is counterproductive and unfair. When Americans believed that fat caused obesity, food companies made many low-fat products. When Americans believed that carbohydrates caused obesity, companies made many low-carb products. If these products had worked better, food companies would have made more of them.

If the Shangri-La diet and the theory behind it have merit, what new products and services might we expect from the food industry, besides the obvious (bottled sugar water and tote-sized ELOO)?

- *More consumer control of flavor.* For example, frozen pizza with ten optional toppings, to be added in creative combinations by the chef— the person who heats it up. The more novel the flavor combinations, the less fattening the food would be. At a movie theater I attended recently, you could flavor your popcorn using twelve different shakers, with flavors such as apple cinnamon, ranch, and chocolate marshmallow.

- *Lots of new flavors.* Mango-mint soda, anyone? A flavor-of-the-month program created by soft-drink companies might work. The new flavors wouldn't be available long enough to become familiar.

- *More slowly digested foods.* This means foods with a lower glycemic index, as discussed in Chapter 6, "Extra Credit: Eight More Ways to Lose Weight." A first step is adding a food's glycemic index to the mandatory nutritional information on the package. Some Australian food manufacturers put something called the GI Symbol (www.gisymbol.com.au) on food labels, along with the food's glycemic index. Cargill, a huge American ingredients company, recently introduced two new sweeteners (one liquid, one powder) whose key property is that they are slowly digested. Because these sweeteners are caloric, they can be used to make sugar water for the Shangri-La diet.

- *Low-flavor foods.* "Half the flavor, all the calories" sounds more sarcastic than appetizing. But low-salt foods are found in every supermarket. Foods with less added flavor than usual may be possible as well, perhaps under the name *delicate-flavor foods.* Delicately flavored foods, even when eaten many times, will raise the set point less than strongly flavored foods.

- *Emphasis on qualities other than flavor.* Foods with weaker flavor-calorie associations taste less good—there is no avoiding this. But Food A may have a weaker flavor-calorie association than Food B, yet still be as pleasant as Food B if Food A is superior to Food B in other ways that bring us pleasure, such as appearance and texture. Sushi is very popular, for instance, yet it usually has a weak flavor. Excellent appearance and texture compensate for the weak flavor. A particularly good take-out pizza store near my house offers only one topping per day. Every day, the topping changes. They reap little benefit from flavor-calorie associations, but their pizza is wildly popular because of its originality, great appearance, great texture, and a certain something that comes from using high-end ingredients.

- *Promote connoisseurship.* Food connoisseurs avoid ditto foods—exactly the foods that my theory says you should avoid. They search out, purchase, eat, and even glorify foods with unusual and subtle flavors—exactly the foods my theory says you should eat. Inevitably these foods are made in small batches and cannot become very familiar. A culture of food connoisseurship may be the main reason that the French are less obese than Americans.

- *Foods that intentionally vary in flavor.* During that fateful trip to Paris (see Chapter 2, "The Case of the Missing Appetite"), I drank ordinary soft drinks and lost weight. They caused weight loss because their flavors were unfamiliar. Could a soda be made whose flavor would *always* be unfamiliar? Yes, if the flavor varied enough from one serving to the next. To produce such a soda would require a new kind of manufacturing. Food companies (and other manufacturers) work hard to ensure that their products are always the same. Quality control in manufacturing means minimizing variation. The goal of this new kind of manufacturing would be to *introduce* variation in a controlled way—enough so that the soda is far less fattening, but not so much that consumers are confused. It is probably impossible to make each bottle different from every other bottle, but the goal would be to introduce enough variation so that the flavor would never become familiar. If the variation were large enough, drinking this newfangled soda would help you lose weight, just as I lost weight in Paris. It would be better than plain sugar water because you could drink it at meals. If you drink *unflavored* sugar water at a meal, it will simply strengthen the flavor-calorie associations of the flavors of the rest of the meal. *Flavored* sugar water will not have this effect. The flavor of the sugar water will interfere with the association of the flavors of other foods and the sugar-water calories.

In recent years, big food companies have clearly been interested in making their product lines healthier. Coca-Cola bought Odwalla, a manufacturer of fruit juices, for exactly that reason. McDonald's introduced more salad variety and put fresh fruit on their menu. What I hope will interest food company executives is the idea that *you can make a weight-loss version of Coke.* This is completely new. It would require substantial innovations in manufacturing, but the potential market for this product and the other products and services I have described is enormous.

The Antidote to Civilization

Club Med, the resort chain, used to call itself "the antidote to civilization"—a brilliant and revealing slogan. It revealed two things: A substantial fraction of the target audience (people rich enough to afford Club Med) was (a) slightly miserable (thus needing an "antidote") and (b) convinced that civilization was the source of their discontent. Club Med offered a vaguely pre-civilized life—for example, outdoor activities, no money—for a week or two.

The obesity epidemic is clearly a by-product of civilization. We don't just have plenty of food; we also have enough money to pay for considerable processing of that food. Proposed solutions to the obesity epidemic have often had a Club Med–like flavor: Outlaw television. Make exercise mandatory. No foods introduced since 1950. These solutions are appealing, alas, for the same reason Club Med is appealing: We believe in our hearts that something is wrong with civilization.

These views are not wrong, exactly, but they are doughnut truths. Something crucial is missing. The urban theorist and author Jane Jacobs had a great way of putting it. In discussing what to do about pollution, she said the problem is not too much this or too little that; the problem is the undone work— by which she meant the intricate, time-consuming development of new ideas and new products and services based on those ideas. The antidote to civilization, Jacobs would say, is more civilization.

A diet book is a low form of civilization. In this chapter, I have indicated what some higher forms might be, including new school curricula and new food products. They are only the beginning. When creative and resourceful people have the right ideas about the causes of obesity, they will begin to change our world in many ways that make it much harder to become obese.

Appendix

THE SCIENCE BEHIND THE THEORY BEHIND THE DIET

"AM I THE only one who thinks this diet might be an enormous hoax perpetrated by the *Freakonomics* guys?" posted someone on a blog about the Shangri-La diet. "I hardly believe it myself," someone replied—someone for whom it was working. They weren't the only ones. After *Good Morning America* ran a piece about it, Diane Sawyer's first words were: "Jaws are dropping around the studio." One reason the diet is so surprising is that it is based on science that most people—including, unfortunately, most obesity researchers—are unaware of.

I would like to change that. You don't need to know about the science to do the diet; that's why this is an appendix. But for those who are interested, here's a brief explanation of the scientific basis for the diet, especially the work of the three scientists—Michel Cabanac, Anthony Sclafani, and Israel Ramirez—who influenced me the most.

Physiology Meets Psychology

The theory behind the Shangri-La diet is based on research in two areas that are usually separate: weight control and associative learning. Most weight-control researchers know little about associative learning, and most associative-learning researchers know little about weight control. The two topics are studied in different university departments: weight control in physiology, associative learning in psychology.

A central concept in physiology is *homeostasis*: the maintenance of constant conditions. Throughout our bodies, homeostasis is happening in hundreds of ways. Sweating when you are hot and shivering when you are cold are ways your brain keeps your body temperature constant. The oil on your skin is another example. Washing your face causes your oil glands to become more active in order to restore the oil you washed away. The concentrations of many substances in your blood, including oxygen and glucose (blood sugar), are kept constant in various ways.

Around 1950, a London researcher named G. Kennedy made observations about the weight of rats that suggested that body fat too was homeostatically regulated. The rats were fed rat chow mixed with water. Kennedy varied how much water was mixed with the chow. When the amount of water was doubled, thus cutting the density of calories in half, for a few days the rats ate fewer calories than usual. As a result, they lost weight. A few days after that, however, they started eating more calories than usual, enough to regain the lost weight. Subsequently, they ate enough each day to stay at their pre-dilution weight. Their weight remained quite constant even when their food changed a lot, just as a thermostat-controlled heating-and-cooling system keeps a room's temperature roughly the same even when the outside temperature changes. Kennedy proposed that a thermostat-like system—in other words, a system with a set point—controls our weight.

Kennedy's proposal was supported by the discovery of the hormone leptin in 1994. In order to regulate the amount of body fat, the brain must be able to know how much body fat you have, just as a thermostat needs a built-in thermometer to keep track of the room temperature. Leptin serves as the brain's body-fat thermometer: The concentration of leptin in your blood tells your brain how much fat is in your body. Leptin is produced by fat cells. When your body fat goes up, so does the amount of leptin in your blood. When your body fat goes down, leptin goes down.

Associative learning is as central to psychology as homeostasis is to physiology. One type of associative learning is Pavlovian conditioning, discovered by Ivan Pavlov, the Russian physiologist. In laboratory experiments, Pavlov found that if he rang a bell for two minutes and then gave a dog food, the dog quickly learned to associate the sound of the bell with arrival of the food. After several of these bell-food pairings, ringing the bell would cause the dog to salivate in anticipation of receiving food.

The generalizations that Pavlov discovered by studying bells, food, and salivation turned out to predict what happens in many other situations. They have helped us understand fear, hunger, food aversions, drug tolerance, drug addiction, sexual arousal, and even visual aftereffects. My graduate training was close to this area of psychology.

Kennedy's set-point theory of weight control and Pavlov's learning experiments are well known. They were the starting points for the science that led to my theory.

Michel Cabanac: The University of Cold Water

Dr. Michel Cabanac is a professor of physiology at Laval University, in Quebec. His first research project, as a medical student in Lyon, France, was about thermoregulation in dogs. After graduation, in 1958, he went to Paris, where his boss assigned him to study thermoregulation in humans. The research involved subjects sitting in a tub of hot water. One day Cabanac himself served as a subject. The hot water made him very warm. Cleaning the equipment afterward, he got some cold water on his hands and he noticed it felt good. "To me this was Newton's apple," he said, referring to the story that a falling apple inspired Newton's theory of gravity. He suddenly had an idea about why we feel pleasure and pain. Part of what makes a temperature feel pleasant or unpleasant, he realized, was a *difference*: the difference between the body's set-point temperature (the temperature the system tries to maintain) and the body's actual (core) temperature. If your core temperature is *higher* than your set point, cold water feels pleasant. That was Cabanac's situation: Sitting in the hot water had raised his core temperature above his set point. But if your core temperature is *lower* than your set point, cold water feels unpleasant. Because we seek and continue pleasant experiences and avoid or end unpleasant ones, these hedonic changes help us regulate our body temperature.

Cabanac wanted to test his idea about pleasure in other domains. Food is another source of pleasure. Do changes in how pleasant we find food help regulate our weight? He began to study what controls how pleasant we find a sip of sugar water. For years, he got nowhere; nothing he tried changed how his subjects responded. He did find that if subjects were given glucose in water through a tube into their stomach, sips of sugar water became less pleasant. This was a whittled-down laboratory version of what happens during a meal: Calories go into your stomach, your body senses the calories, food becomes less pleasant (and when it reaches "not pleasant," you stop eating). Just as the pleasantness of cold water depends on the difference between set-point temperature and core temperature, Cabanac believed that the pleasantness of sweet water would depend on the difference between body-weight set point and actual weight.

To test this prediction, he did an experiment in which subjects lost eight pounds by eating less of their usual food. This was meant to lower their actual weight below their set point. He was one of the subjects. He told me, "It was torture. You dream you are breaking the fast and ruining the experiment." At the lower weight, glucose water sent directly into the stomach through a tube no longer reduced how pleasant sips of sweet water tasted. A force that pushes people to stop eating—the food stops tasting good—was no longer present. Cabanac concluded that when your weight is below your set point, it takes more food to feel full. Implicit in this was the prediction that when your weight is *above* your set point, it will take *less* food to feel full.

Cabanac's experiment came to life for me when countless Shangri-La dieters spoke of needing much less food to feel full. "This is the first time I have ever left food on a plate at a meal," wrote one. "I'm able to feel full after eating about half of what I normally eat," wrote another. I had had the same experience. These comments were an excellent sign that the Shangri-La diet works as I theorized: It lowers your set point.

Cabanac did another experiment to see if the "laws" of temperature regulation applied to weight regulation. In temperature regulation, skin temperature affects the set point. Warming the skin lowers the body temperature set point; cooling the skin raises the set point. "This anticipates future threat," said Cabanac. The key idea is that the set point is sensitive to prevailing conditions in the outside world.

To see if something similar happened with weight, Cabanac and a colleague did an experiment in which participants got all their calories from what Cabanac called "a very flat food," a bland liquid diet. The subjects, one of whom was Cabanac, could eat as much of the liquid diet as they wanted, but they still lost weight, as Cabanac had predicted. In contrast to calorie restriction ("torture"), this way of losing weight was "painless," said Cabanac. "The subjects, including myself, lost and lost and lost weight and did not suffer. Without feeling hungry—never." The experiment continued until they had lost as much weight as the participants in the earlier calorie-restriction experiment. Then, while the subjects were at their lower weight, the glucose-loading test was repeated. This time the results were perfectly normal: The glucose load in the stomach made sips of the sweet water taste less pleasant. Cabanac's explanation is that in this case the weight loss did not change the results because set point and actual weight stayed close. When you lose weight by eating bland food (easy), your set point goes down. When you lose weight by calorie restriction (hard), your set point doesn't go down. That there are two quite different ways of losing weight—with and without set-point reduction—is a very important idea.

The bland-food experiment also impressed me because it demonstrated with human subjects that your set point depends on what you eat. Unfortunately, Cabanac's work didn't receive the attention it deserved. When I asked him what the rest of the world made of it, he said he didn't think it had been cited at all in other professional publications. He checked, however, and found that it had been cited twenty times since publication in 1976—not much, considering the vast interest in weight loss.

Around the same time as the bland-food experiment, a student in Cabanac's lab named Marc Fantino, who is now a medical school professor in Dijon, France, did a similar but more extreme experiment, in which four subjects got all of their nutrition via a tube through the nose into the stomach—nutrition without any flavor at all, in other words. They could consume as much as they wanted but lost weight quickly, quite a bit faster than the subjects in the bland-food experiment, even though the food was the same. This suggested to me that flavor raised the set point. Without any flavor, the set point went down quickly.

Surely, I thought, some flavors were more potent than others. What did you need to know about a flavor to predict *how much* it would increase the set point? Cabanac's and Fantino's research raised this question but did not help answer it.

Anthony Sclafani: Why We Like Spinach

Dr. Anthony Sclafani is a professor of psychology at Brooklyn College, a branch of the City University of New York. In the 1970s, he was looking for an animal model of obesity. It is surprisingly hard to make normal rats fat. At the time, the usual way of making rats fat was to add fat to their chow by mixing in a solid shortening, such as Crisco. This produced obesity, but slowly. Maybe if the food tasted better, they would get fat more quickly, reasoned Sclafani. He sent one of his graduate students to the supermarket and had him bring back fattening foods such as sweetened condensed milk, chocolate-chip cookies, salami, cheese, bananas, marshmallows, milk chocolate, and peanut butter.

When young, still-growing rats were given these foods in addition to rat chow, they gained weight more than twice as fast as when given only rat chow, and much faster than rats given a high-fat diet. This suggested that supermarket food was quite fattening compared to rat chow, and that it was not just its high fat content that made it fattening. This research was published in the same year

(1976) and journal (*Physiology & Behavior*) as Cabanac's bland-food experiment, separated by just a few hundred pages. Both experiments—rat (Sclafani), human (Cabanac), weight gain (Sclafani), weight loss (Cabanac)—suggested to me that the flavor of food controls the set point. Good-tasting food raises the set point; not-so-good-tasting food lowers it.

Ten years later, Sclafani was still studying food intake. By accident, he had discovered that rats have a remarkable appetite for a partially digested starch called Polycose. To humans this is a bland source of calories; if you add it to orange juice, it doesn't change the flavor. But rats loved it. This attractiveness had a curious quality: It increased over days. For example, rats initially preferred sugar water to Polycose water, but over a period of several days switched their preference to the Polycose solution. This suggested to Sclafani that Polycose had powerful effects *after* ingestion that caused its taste to become very attractive. The notion that flavors become better tasting when they are associated with calories or nutrients that are detected by the digestive system had been kicking around since the 1960s. But there had been only a few demonstrations of such learning and in those cases the learning had been weak.

Maybe, thought Sclafani, the question—*Does flavor–calorie associative learning really exist?*—was worth revisiting. Sclafani and a colleague set up an apparatus that would inject either Polycose water or plain water directly into a rat's stomach whenever it drank. The experiment used two flavors of Kool-Aid. When a rat drank water with Flavor 1, it got Polycose water injected into its stomach. When it drank water with Flavor 2, it got plain water injected into its stomach. In contrast to the weak effects of earlier research, this procedure produced a huge preference for water with Flavor 1 when the rat was given a choice between the two flavors. Even after the Polycose injections were stopped and both Kool-Aid flavors were followed by injections of plain water, the preference persisted for days.

Sclafani hadn't discovered flavor-calorie learning; earlier researchers had done that. What he *had* done was discover its importance, its power, and how to study it. In the following years, Sclafani and his colleagues did hundreds of experiments about flavor-calorie learning. They made it real. By the time I started theorizing about weight control, it was so firmly established that I took it for granted.

Israel Ramirez: Connecting Associative Learning and Weight Control

When Dr. Israel Ramirez worked at the Monell Chemical Senses Institute, in Philadelphia (1982–1997), he did one brilliant experiment after another. Psychology and physiology research is intensely empirical. Everything revolves around data, usually from experiments. Compared to other scientists who study food intake, Cabanac is a great theorist whose experiments deftly support his theoretical ideas, and Sclafani is a great empiricist whose experiments make a rich pointillist picture of an empirical generalization. Ramirez was a Shakespearean court jester type of scientist whose experiments obliquely spoke deep truths.

On the face of it, Ramirez was a scientist whose specialty was doing experiments with hard-to-explain results. This is a difficult position for a scientist. Puzzling results are the most enlightening, or at least they can be, but it may take quite a while to figure out the explanation, and in the meantime the value of your work is unclear. Ramirez single-handedly gave the whole field of weight control a big push forward, but it was not obvious at the time.

Ramirez is now a software consultant and developer at PC Helps Support, Bala Cynwd, Pennsylvania. He did so much great work at Monell that when I interviewed him in 2005 he did not remember an outstanding review paper he had written twenty years earlier about whether sugar causes obesity. "It is widely believed," the paper began, "that consumption of sucrose may predispose human beings to obesity." Ramirez concluded, however, that "animal [rat] studies do not support [this] idea." He pointed out that sugar has a much different effect on weight when it is eaten "wet" (dissolved in water) than when eaten dry. This is not consistent with the simple idea that sugar is fattening. Because rats and humans are quite similar in many dietary ways, this was powerful evidence against the conventional view.

After Sclafani commented that rats given bread in addition to their regular chow became obese, Ramirez decided to do a simple experiment. He compared two groups of rats given bread as their only source of calories. One group got ordinary bread mix modified so that it was nutritionally complete. The other group got the same mix in the form of actual bread, which was made by adding water to the mix and baking it. Thus the two groups were offered the same nutrients, the same micronutrients, the same proportions of fat, carbohydrate, and protein. After several weeks, the rats given cooked bread weighed substantially more than the rats given bread mix. The experiment is so simple and easy that a seventh-grader could do it, yet it shows that something important is missing from conventional weight-control ideas. "It was an ugly sort of thing," he told me. (In fact, it was beautifully simple, both in thought and execution. By "ugly" Ramirez meant it was hard to say exactly how the cooked bread differed from the uncooked bread.) When he told colleagues about it, "it evoked a bit of laughter." He didn't publish it.

He did think about it, though. One difference between the bread mix and the bread was the water added to make the bread. So Ramirez did several experiments that measured the effect of adding water to dry rat chow. They showed that water was fattening—very fattening! Young rats given wet food gained more weight than rats given dry food, even though both groups had water available from a water bottle. The effect was huge: The right amount of water could *double* the rats' weight gain. This contradicts everything the average American has been told about weight control. Dieters are always told to drink lots of water, because water has no calories, no fat, no carbohydrate, no sugar, no anything. When I tell people this result they are usually dumbfounded. Ramirez himself was unsure how to explain it. My theory, however, explains this astonishing result because it is likely that moistening the chow both increased its flavor and speeded up its digestion, thereby leading to stronger flavor-calorie associations.

Sclafani's flavor-calorie learning experiments demonstrated something that many others had believed but had been unable to show. Cabanac's experiments were beautiful demonstrations that exposed a hidden logic already known to Cabanac. Ramirez's experiments, on the other hand, usually exposed everyone's *lack* of understanding, including his own.

One set of Ramirez's experiments went further. Like so many important discoveries, it began with a kind of accident. Along the lines of the bread experiment, Ramirez was wondering how to cause "overeating" without changing macronutrient (fat/protein/carbohydrate) composition. Farmers had tried adding saccharin to livestock feed in order to fatten their animals more quickly. Maybe the saccharin would make the food taste better so the animals would eat more of it. As far as Ramirez knew, this had always failed. But maybe it was worth another try.

The experimental design was simple: He used two groups of rats. Both groups were given a liquid diet (the diet needed to be liquid so that the saccharin could be added). One group got the liquid diet with saccharin; the other group got the liquid diet without saccharin. The first two experiments gave inconsistent results. In one Ramirez got an effect (the rats given saccharin ate more and gained more weight), in the other he didn't. "[A colleague] was looking at my results," Ramirez said. "He thought it was silly: Half were successful, half weren't."

Ramirez assumed that the reason for the inconsistent results was that some rats naturally liked saccharin and some did not. If he could sort the rats into those two groups—those that liked saccharin and those that didn't—the results should become strong and clear. The rats that liked saccharin would gain weight, and the ones that didn't like it would not. So he did an experiment in which he measured how much each rat liked saccharin before going on to measure the effect of saccharin on each rat's weight.

This experiment had a curious result: Saccharin had no effect. The weights of the two groups did not differ. Yet the only difference between this experiment and an earlier experiment where saccharin *did* have an effect was the saccharin-preference test at the beginning. Ramirez had assumed that the preference test itself would not affect the rats' weight. Preference tests are harmless, right? If someone asks you how much you like chocolate, surely that does not make chocolate any less fattening. If you fill out a three-page survey about hot dogs, surely that does not make the hot dogs you eat less fattening. The saccharin preference test had consisted of giving rats a bottle of saccharin-flavored water in their home cage (in addition to plain water) for four days. The rats that drank the most saccharin-flavored water were assumed to like saccharin the most. Surely such an innocuous experience would not affect the rats' weight. But it did. A new experiment, in which some rats were given the preference test and others were not, showed this conclusively.

One way to think about the results was this: Only if the saccharin was *new* would adding it to the liquid diet make that diet more fattening. If the saccharin was familiar, it did not make the liquid diet more fattening. Ramirez looked at the earlier experiment that had failed to find an effect of saccharin. In that experiment, the rats had gotten the liquid diet for one week before the saccharin was added. This suggested that the *liquid diet* must also be new when it is combined with saccharin for the saccharin to be effective. All in all, the experiments suggested that *experience* with a food affected how fattening it was. That is one of the key ideas of my weight-control theory. At the end of the scientific paper about these results, Ramirez wrote that "the present report provides the first evidence that learning may be an important factor in dietary hyperphagia [overeating]."

Indeed it did. This was a radical new idea. Apparently no one who read the paper knew what to make of it. It was rarely cited. "You picked up on it," Ramirez told me in 2005. "No one else did."

Because of my graduate training in psychology, I knew a lot about Pavlovian conditioning. That the saccharin and the liquid diet both had to be new to the rats in order to get the effect immediately suggested to me that Pavlovian conditioning was involved; more specifically, it suggested that the effect was due to a *learned association* between the flavor of the saccharin and the calories of the liquid diet. Because of Sclafani's work, I took it for granted that such learning happened. Because of Cabanac's work, I assumed that anything that increased weight did so by raising the set point. Cabanac and Sclafani had persuasively demonstrated that what you eat, especially its flavor, can influence your body-weight set point, so it was easy to believe that flavor-calorie associations affected the set point.

There was a little more to my new theory than that, but not much.

For more about the science behind the theory, see www.sethroberts.net/articles/whatmakesfood fattening.pdf.

ACKNOWLEDGMENTS

IF MY Croatian friend Jasmina Kos had not invited me to visit her, causing me to spend a week in Paris . . . thanks, Jasmina. Carl Willat has been endlessly helpful and encouraging, including the curious suggestion that this book be circle shaped and titled *You Look Like This*. "Help it stand out," he said.

I am grateful to the many friends who tried my weight-loss methods and told their friends about them. Their experiences were the first signs that these ideas could help many people. My students have been a cheerful and inquisitive audience and have had a way of testing my ideas without telling me, which I found quite complimentary.

For help with the research behind this book, I

want to thank Janessa Karawan, who continued to assist me even after she got a full-time job because she thought it was such an interesting project; Katie Kelly, who helped in many ways; and my mother, Justine Roberts (a medical librarian). My mom, who knew all about database searches long before Google—when they were called *queries*—did hundreds of them to help me out.

I thank Margaret Adamek, Elizabeth Capaldi, David Cutler, William Jacobs, Frances Jalet-Miller, Naomi Katz, Inas Rashad (who also helped with Figure 7), Paul Rozin, and Norman Temple for speaking with me. Michel Cabanac, Antonia Demas, Israel Ramirez, and Anthony Sclafani (who also gave me a tour of his lab) each spent several hours answering my questions. In the Appendix I try to explain how important the work of Cabanac, Ramirez, and Sclafani has been to my thinking. Israel Ramirez talked to me at length ten years ago, too. My theory of weight control was inspired by one of the twenty-odd reprints of his papers that he sent me back then.

That was before open access (free availability of research via the Web). The combination of open access and blogs did wonders for this book. Stevan Harnad has not only pushed for open access for many years, but he also founded *Behavioral and Brain Sciences*, where the scientific article behind this book was published, built it into a highly cited open-access journal, and was the editor who accepted my article. I am very grateful to Andrew Gelman, a longtime friend, who wrote about my work at www.stat.columbia.edu/~gelman/blog. Open access meant readers of his blog could read my article and see for themselves. His comments drew the attention of Alex Tabarrok at the Marginal Revolution (www.marginalrevolution.com), who wrote the most favorable notice my work has ever received.

Stephen Dubner and Steven Levitt, the authors of *Freakonomics*, learned about my work via Marginal Revolution, and drew it to the attention of the book industry, not to mention the general public, via a column in the *New York Times*. Not only did they try my ideas themselves, but they also invited me to guest-blog at www.freakonomics.com. That led Ann Hendricks to set up a blog where people trying the Shangri-La diet—the bootleg version—could swap stories. Their stories and enthusiasm made writing this book much easier, as I mentioned in the Introduction.

My agent, Suzanne Gluck, as she so often does, did a great job of generating interest among publishers; whenever something good happens related to this book, I call it "the Gluck effect." Laura Bellotti helped me prepare a proposal and sample chapters that Suzanne had very little quarrel with.

"Everyone needs an editor," says a friend of mine. I need an editor more than most—thank goodness Marian Lizzi, my editor at Putnam, was there for me. When I was unsure about what to do— and this happened a lot—I would phone Marian and ask. I'm a little amazed how often I agreed with her suggestions. Helping me write the book, Sheila Buff provided a good sounding board, much-needed health expertise, and cogent advice.

"The diet book with a Ph.D.," Marian has wittily called it. My Ph.D. is in experimental psychology, and in several ways this is the sort of book an experimental psychologist would write (e.g., taking experiments with rats seriously). I have learned more experimental psychology from Saul Sternberg, a research scientist at Bell Labs and a professor at the University of Pennsylvania, than from anyone else. He has been incredibly supportive throughout my academic career. When I was a graduate student, Saul invited me to give a talk at Bell Labs. Afterward, we had dinner at his house. There was a graph of some data on the refrigerator. "What's this?" I asked. "The force of gravity," he said. It was a graph of his weight.

In the afterword to *Exploratory Data Analysis* (1977), a great statistics book, John Tukey wrote that he hadn't mentioned computers in the main text but their shadow fell on every page. This book is dedicated to animal-learning researchers because my debt to them is no less than Tukey's to computers. They built up a body of work, thousands of experiments about associative learning and how to study it, without which this book would never have been possible.

My friend William Rubel, author of *The Magic of Fire* (about hearth cooking), suggested having Internet forums for the book. What great advice that was!

NOTES

Abbreviations

Annie's blog: www.blogger.com/comment.g?blogID
=16962289&postID=112729758775514780

CalorieLab blog: http://calorielab.com/news/2005
/09/21/ seth-roberts-shangri-la-diet-in-detail

Epigraph

ix "Curiously enough, the immense dinner . . . hungrier than usual": Nancy Mitford, *Love in a Cold Climate* (New York: Modern Library, 1994), 339.

Introduction

2 when I wrote for *Spy* magazine: Seth Roberts, "Lab Rat: What AIDS Researcher Dr. Robert Gallo Did in Pursuit of the Nobel Prize, and What

He Didn't Do in Pursuit of a Cure for AIDS," *Spy*, June 1990, 70–79. Available at www.virusmyth .net/aids/data/srlabrat.htm, accessed December 15, 2005.

3   "The common aim of all science . . . the gradual removal of prejudices": Niels Bohr, *Atomic Physics and Human Knowledge* (New York: John Wiley Science Editions, 1961), 31.

Chapter 1. Why a Calorie Is Not a Calorie

5   One of the guys said to the other . . . a one-pound box of candy and gain 10 pounds": Mary Kate Norton, "Men Are Pigs," *The Daily Californian*, July 25, 2000, 3.

5   the term *doughnut truth* to mean "only the truth, and the whole truth, with a hole in the truth": Vladimir Nabokov, *Ada* (New York: McGraw-Hill, 1969), 154.

6   Everything should be about portion size: Marion Nestle comment during the "Table for Twelve," segment of *On the Media* (WNYC), April 22, 2005. Transcript at www.onthemedia.org/transcripts/ transcripts_042205_food.html, accessed January 5, 2005.

17   He later wrote it tasted "like medicine": Gaku Homma, *The Folk Art of Japanese Country Cooking* (Berkeley, Calif.: North Atlantic Books, 1991), 21.

17   "First put off by the leaves' flavor, after repeated exposure I grew to anticipate their taste":

Jonathan Kauffman, "A Star Is Stewed," *East Bay Express,* October 6, 2004. At www
.eastbayexpress.com/Issues/2004-10-06/dining/
food__print.html, accessed December 9, 2005.

Chapter 2. The Case of the Missing Appetite

21 This new, $3 billion-a-year industry was aimed squarely at . . . never works: Margaret Webb Pressler, "Low-Carb Fad Fades, and Atkins Is Big Loser," *The Washington Post*, August 2, 2005, A01.

26 There was no precedent anywhere . . . causing so much weight loss: For more about my weight-loss self-experimentation, see Seth Roberts, "Self-experimentation as a Source of New Ideas: Ten Examples About Sleep, Mood, Health, and Weight," *Behavioral and Brain Sciences* 27 (2) (April 2004): 227–288. Available at http://repositories.cdlib.org/postprints/117.

29 "There is something unpleasant or aversive about sweetness when food deprivation is high" . . . based on her research: Elizabeth D. Capaldi, "Conditioned Food Preferences," in Elizabeth D. Capaldi, ed., *Why We Eat What We Eat: The Psychology of Eating* (Washington, D.C.: American Psychological Association, 1996). Quotation from p. 67.

31 Olive oil is a staple of the Mediterranean diet, eaten by Italians, Greeks . . . have low rates of heart disease: Walter C. Willett et al.

"Mediterranean Diet Pyramid: A Cultural Model for Healthy Eating," *American Journal of Clinical Nutrition* 61, Suppl. 6 (June 1995): 1402S–1406S. Chapter 4 of *Eat, Drink, and Be Healthy: The Harvard Medical School Guide to Healthy Eating* (New York: Simon & Schuster, 2002), by Walter Willett, describes other reasons to think olive oil is healthy.

32 My metabolism had slowed down: Experiments with rats and humans have shown that your metabolism slows down. For example, see Jules Hirsch, Lisa C. Hudgins, Rudolph L. Leibel, and Michael Rosenbaum, "Diet Composition and Energy Balance in Humans," *American Journal of Clinical Nutrition* 67, Suppl. 3 (1998): 551S–555S.

33 According to *New Yorker* writer Malcolm Gladwell, diet books "have an unspoken set of narrative rules and conventions . . . the radical truth that inspired his diet": Malcolm Gladwell, "The Pima Paradox," *The New Yorker*, February 2, 1998. Available at www.gladwell.com/1998/1998_02_02_a_pima.htm, accessed January 27, 2006.

35 "Weight loss is not for the fainthearted," said Dr. Thomas Wadden . . . in 2005: Gina Kolata, "Diet and Lose Weight? Scientists Say 'Prove It!,' " *The New York Times*, January 4, 2005.

Interlude. Never This Thin

37 Interviews on October 12, 2006, and December
    11, 2006, posts at http://boards.sethroberts.net/
    index.php?topic=2698.msg21470#msg21470 and
    http://boards.sethroberts.net/index.php?topic=
    2698.msg24905#msg24905.

Interlude. Life Regained

50 http://ethesis.blogspot.com/search/label/
    Shangri-la%20Diet, interviews on September 14,
    2006, and December 10, 2006, a fax on December
    10, 2006, and e-mail on December 13, 2006.

Chapter 4. How to Do the Shangri-La Diet

52 Secretly, I suspected the answer to weight is-
    sues would be something ridiculously simple,
    but this is almost too much to hope for: Emily
    Jones, "Another Venture into La La Land,"
    Starkville Daily News, November 16, 2005. At
    http://starkvilledailynews.com/articles/2005/11
    /16/news/lifestyles/lifestyles02, accessed No-
    vember 21, 2005.

52 It appealed to my essential laziness: CalorieLab
    blog/#comment-743 (Leftblanc, posted Nov-
    ember 25, 2005), accessed November 25, 2005.

58 Omega-3: Not Overrated, pp. 58–61: Susan
    Allport, *The Queen of Fats* (Berkeley: University
    of California Press, 2006); Christine M. Albert, et
    al., "Blood levels of long-chain n-3 fatty acids
    and the risk of sudden death," *New England*

Journal of Medicine 346 (2002):1113–18; Simona Noaghuil, et al., "Cross-national comparisons of seafood consumption and rates of bipolar disorders," *American Journal of Psychiatry* 160 (2003): 2222–27; Gordon Parker, et al., "Omega-3 fatty acids and mood disorders," *American Journal of Psychiatry* 163 (2006): 969–78; Martha Clare Innis, et al., "Fish consumption and cognitive decline with age in a large community study," *Archives of Neurology* 62 (2005): 1849–53.

59 A well-known clinical trial called the Lyon Diet Heart Study . . . one heart attack: Michel de Lorgeril et al., "Mediterranean Diet, Traditional Risk Factors, and the Rate of Cardiovascular Complications After Myocardial Infarction: Final Report of the Lyon Diet Heart Study," *Circulation* 99 (6) (February 16, 1999): 779–85.

60 Israeli paradox: Susan Allport, "The skinny on fat," *Gastronomica* (Winter 2003), 3 no. 1, 28–36. Available online on December 15, 2006, at http://caliber.ucpress.net/doi/pdf/10.1525/gfc.2003.3.1.28?cookieSet=1.

61 omega-6/omega-3 ratios: Artemis P. Simopoulos, "The importance of the ratio of omega-6/omega-3 essential fatty acids," *Biomedical Pharmacotherapeutics* (2002) 56 no. 8:365–79. For a good overview of why omega-6 is dangerous, see www.health-heart.org/poster.pdf.

62 fewer menstrual headaches: http://boards.sethroberts.net/index.php?topic=3437.0

62 reduction of arthritis: http://boards.sethroberts
    .net/index.php?topic=678.0

62 reduction of rosacea: http://boards.sethroberts
    .net/index.php?topic=3433.msg30832#msg30832

62 1971 study: M. L. Pearce, et al., "Incidence of
    cancer in men on a diet high in polyunsaturated
    fat," *Lancet* (March 6, 1971), 1 no. 7697: 464–67.

64 Dr. William Jacobs is a professor of psychiatry
    at the University of Florida's College of
    Medicine . . . Overeating and Eating Disorders
    Clinic: Interview with William Jacobs,
    November 21, 2005.

65 One set found that a flavor-calorie association . . .
    eating the calorie source: Elizabeth D. Capaldi
    et al., "Conditioned Flavor Preferences Based
    on Delayed Caloric Consequences," *Journal of
    Experimental Psychology: Animal Behavior
    Processes* 13 (2) (April 1987): 150–55.

65 The other set found that a one-hour interval . . .
    from being learned: Robert A. Boakes and Todd
    Lubart, "Enhanced Preference for a Flavour
    Following Reversed Flavour/Glucose Pairing,"
    *Quarterly Journal of Experimental Psychology
    B: Comparative and Physiological Psychology* 40
    (1, Sec. B) (February 1988): 49–62.

66 "I ate *pesto* yesterday": Annie's blog (Masa'il,
    posted October 3, 2005), accessed November
    21, 2005.

67 "Tried this diet for 2 days and I am not as hun-
    gry . . . Unbelievable": www.chowhound.com/
    boards/notfood/messages/64541.html (Adfasf,

posted November 16, 2005), accessed November 19, 2005.

67 "This is the first time I have ever left food on a plate": www.freakonomics.com/blog/2005/09/09/freakonomics-in-the-ny-times-the-shangri-la-diet/#comments (Jnyc, posted September 18, 2005), accessed November 19, 2005.

67 "I'm able to feel full after eating about half of what I normally eat": www.freakonomics.com/blog/2005/09/09/freakonomics-in-the-ny-times-the-shangri-la-diet/#comments (Anonymous, posted September 20, 2005), accessed November 21, 2005.

68 "I was a three slices guy; now one slice of pizza is enough": CalorieLab blog/#comment-743 (Leftblanc, posted November 25, 2005), accessed November 25, 2005.

68 "I went to a buffet . . . really bloated afterward," wrote one Shangri-La dieter: Annie's blog (Molly, posted October 1, 2005), accessed November 21, 2005.

68 "I would wake up and crave something to eat . . . through the night, never": e-mail from RJ, November 18, 2005.

68 "I have gotten the best sleep in I can't tell you how long": e-mail from RJ, November 18, 2005.

69 "I would say I'm not going to eat something sweet . . . than the food is in control of me": Interview with DD, November 8, 2005.

69 "It's true that 400 or 500 calories": Calorie Lab blog/#comment-743 (Leftblanc, posted November 25, 2005), accessed November 25, 2005.

71 "I still have a lot of mouth-boredom/antsiness": Annie's blog (Masa'il, posted September 30, 2005), accessed November 23, 2005.

73 Other Diets at the Same Time, pp. 73–74; interview with Terri Hill, December 6, 2006.

Interlude. End of a Nightmare

75 Interview with Catherine Johnson, November 27, 2006; e-mail from her December 8, 2006; interview with Dr. Erika Schwartz, December 1, 2006.

Chapter 5. Common Questions

83 My emotional eating: http://boards.sethroberts .net/index.php?topic=2319.msg18993#msg18993

83 Emotional eating is: http://boards.sethroberts .net/index.php?topic=2826.msg22875#msg22875

83 When I've gotten: http://boards.sethroberts.net/ index.php?topic=2246.msg18329#msg18329

Interlude. In Shangri-La

84 But here, at Shangri-La, all was in deep calm: James Hilton, *Lost Horizon* (New York: William Morrow, 1933), 142.

84 "Before this, I felt powerless over food": Conversation with DD, November 8, 2005.

84 "It's great to feel like I'm in control of things": Conversation with CM, October 1, 2005.

84 "I never eat the sweets at lunch anymore": Conversation with DD, November 8, 2005.

84 "I can't believe": http://boards.sethroberts .net/index.php?topic=2187.msg18205#msg 18205

85 "[My] weight gain over the years had little to do with being hungry": e-mail from DS, November 14, 2005.

85 "I saw the segment on *GMA* . . . this morning": www.chowhound.com/boards/notfood/messages/ 64520.html (Laura, posted November 14, 2005) accessed November 19, 2005.

85 "The most enormous difference I can see": e-mail from LJ, August 12, 2005.

85 "I like cookies, and they are available at work": groups.expo.st/art/rec.sport.swimming/ 5257 (Martin S., posted September 27, 2005), accessed November 16, 2005.

86 "I used to snack all day": Annie's blog (Leftblanc, posted September 30, 2005), accessed November 19, 2005.

86 "My interest in chocolate has dropped dramatically": Conversation with CM, November 2, 2005.

86 "I just love": http://boards.sethroberts.net/ index.php?topic=1878.msg14808#msg14808

86 "Since I have been doing this, my between-meal cravings have all disappeared": Annie's blog (De

Benci, posted November 15, 2005), accessed
November 19, 2005.

86 "It's just amazing how much my desire to
snack has gone down": Conversation with SC,
December 15, 2005.

87 "I didn't realize to what extent my nighttime
cravings were taking over": Conversation with
CW, November 16, 2005.

87 "The best part of it is the snacking is cut out":
Conversation with BH, December 6, 2005.

87 "I essentially cut all starches out of my diet permanently": Annie's blog (Molly, posted October
5, 2005), accessed November 19, 2005.

87 "My weakness before the program was junky
carbs": Annie's blog (SFD, posted November 15,
2005), accessed November 19, 2005.

87 "A few weeks ago I would have made a beeline
[to the new Starbucks]": Annie's blog (Masa'il,
posted September 30, 2005), accessed December
6, 2005.

87 "This Thursday will make 1 full week since I've
tried it": www.freakonomics.com/blog/2005/
09/09/freakonomics-in-the-ny-times-the-shangri-
la-diet/#comments (Anonymous, posted September 20, 2005), accessed November 19, 2005.

88 "I started [six days ago]": www.freakonomics
.com/blog/2005/09/09/freakonomics-in-the-ny-
times-the-shangri-la-diet/#comments (Jnyc,
posted September 18, 2005), accessed November
19, 2005.

88 "I had a": http://boards.sethroberts.net/index
.php?topic=2807.msg23370#msg23370

88 "I have used the oil for a week now": CalorieLab
blog/#comment-730 (Tina, posted November 22,
2005), accessed November 22, 2005.

88 "Last week a neighbor dropped off a piece of
chocolate cake": CalorieLab blog/#comment-
743 (Leftblanc, posted November 25, 2005), accessed November 25, 2005.

88 "[Before this diet, I] would sometimes wake up
at midnight and eat": Annie's blog (SFC, posted
November 15, 2005), accessed November
19, 2005.

89 "I became a night eater": e-mail from RJ,
November 18, 2005.

89 "I like to measure time by how long it takes to
finish a box of Yodels": Conversation with JC,
October 25, 2005.

89 "The diet works, it's easy, I eat whatever I feel
like": CalorieLab blog/#comment-737 (Leftblanc,
posted November 23, 2005), accessed November
23, 2005.

89 "After a week": http://boards.sethroberts.net/
index.php?topic=2214.msg18995#msg18995

89 "No more late-night snacking": Annie's blog
(Leftblanc, posted September 30, 2005), accessed December 10, 2005.

90 "The constant thoughts I have about eating
have subsided": e-mail from MS, October
27, 2005.

90 "I'm eating to live rather than the other way around": Annie's blog (Molly, posted September 30, 2005), accessed November 22, 2005.

90 "I'm so grateful for not thinking about food all the time": Conversation with DS, November 22, 2005.

90 "I have been able to stop thinking about food": CalorieLab blog/#comment-730 (Tina, posted November 22, 2005), accessed November 22, 2005.

90 "When I do decide to eat, I chose things that are good for me": Annie's blog (Rena, posted December 5, 2005), accessed December 10, 2005.

90 "I am able to make good decisions about how much I need": Annie's blog (Emily, posted December 8, 2005), accessed December 11, 2005.

90 "[Before this diet] I would say I'm not going to eat something sweet": Conversation with DD, November 8, 2005.

91 "I was seeing food as a negative thing because I kept gaining weight": Conversation with CM, October 1, 2005.

91 "When I eat sweets I enjoy it so much more—I savor it": Conversation with DD, October 10, 2005.

Chapter 6. Extra Credit: Eight More Ways to Lose Weight

96 In *French Women Don't Get Fat*: Mireille Guiliano, *French Women Don't Get Fat* (New York: Knopf, 2004), 5.

97 "French women eat dessert three times a day [at cafés] and they're still thin": Dorie Greenspan, author of *Paris Sweets,* interviewed on *To the Best of Our Knowledge,* February 15, 2004. Available at www.wpr.org/book/030209a.html, accessed December 10, 2005.

97 "I think we can say . . . fall outside the Shangri-La Diet": CalorieLab blog/#comment-684, accessed December 10, 2005.

98 *The Flavor Point Diet*: David L. Katz, *The Flavor Point Diet* (New York: Rodale, 2005).

99 "I've been having granola and soy milk for breakfast every day for months . . . Now I'm hungry within a couple of hours": Annie's blog (Jennifer, posted November 20, 2005), accessed November 20, 2005.

100 "The most successful dieters, we've found," wrote Dr. Arthur Agatston in *The South Beach Diet*, . . . a new soup made with every green vegetable he could find": Arthur Agatston, *The South Beach Diet* (New York: Rodale Books, 2003), 43.

100 Yet the husband and wife both drank a lot of Pepsi every day, calling themselves "Pepsiholics":

Susan Sheehan, "Ain't No Middle Class," *The New Yorker*, December 11, 1995, 82–92.

100 "I wasn't wanton with my money . . . to splurge on the extra candy bar, the jumbo Coke": Jill Ciment, *Half a Life* (New York: Crown, 1996), 131.

101 When In-N-Out Burger . . . first customer was a college student majoring in health education: Ed Pope, "New Burger in Town," *San Jose Mercury News*, September 7, 1996, 1A.

101 Dr. William Jacobs, a professor of psychiatry . . . again, all ditto foods: Interview with William Jacobs, November 21, 2005.

102 Dr. Alan Hirsch, a Chicago neurologist, did a study that suggests this will work: Alan R. Hirsch and Mary Beth Gallant-Shean, "Use of Tastants to Facilitate Weight Loss," paper presented at the fifty-third annual meeting of the American Society of Bariatric Physicians, 2004.

104 It has an odd name: *food combining.* Typical food combining rules: www.internethealth library.com/DietandLifestyle/Food_combining .htm, accessed November 20, 2005.

105 An Italian friend of mine went to a diet expert . . . one type of food per meal: Conversation with AF, November 20, 2005.

106 *The New Glucose Revolution:* Jennie Brand-Miller, Thomas M. S. Wolever, Kaye Foster-Powell, and Stephen Colagiuri, *The New Glucose Revolution*, rev. ed. (New York: Marlowe & Company, 2003) .

107 "I just leave off some salt, sweetener or sauce": Annie's blog (Sarah, posted September 30, 2005), accessed November 21, 2005.

108 Timothy Beneke, an Oakland, California, writer, used this idea in a new way: http://timothy beneke.blogspot.com/2005/09/taste-celibacy .html, accessed November 19, 2005; interview with Beneke November 11, 2006; e-mail from Beneke, January 15, 2007.

111 I asked SLD Forums readers: http://boards .sethroberts.net/index.php?topic=3338.0.

Interlude. The Blogosphere Tries It

113 After a *Freakonomics* column about the Shangri-La diet appeared: Stephen J. Dubner and Steven D. Levitt, "Does the Truth Lie Within?" *The New York Times Magazine* (September 11, 2005), 20–22. Available at www.sethroberts.net, accessed December 16, 2005.

113 "I tried a tablespoon of extra-virgin olive oil yesterday": www.freakonomics.com/blog/2005/ 09/13/seth-roberts-guest-blogger-part-ii (Hal, posted September 13, 2005), accessed January 4, 2006.

113 "I don't need to lose weight but I must say this sugar water stuff works": www.freako nomics. com/blog/2005/09/13/seth-roberts-guest-blogger-part-ii (Velopismo, posted September 14, 2005), accessed January 4, 2006.

113 "Whoa. Close to zero appetite": www.freako nomics.com/blog/2005/09/13/seth-roberts-guest-

blogger-part-ii (Molly, posted September 15, 2005), accessed January 4, 2006.

113 "I've lost 6 lbs. in 5 days, despite eating better than I have in years": www.freakonomics .com/blog/2005/09/18/final-guest-blog-from-seth-roberts (Anonymous, posted September 20, 2005), accessed January 27, 2006.

114 "When I started this, I weighed 226": www.freakonomics.com/blog/2005/09/16/seth-roberts-guest-blogger-finale (Anonymous, posted September 21, 2005), accessed January 27, 2006.

114 "I've lost about 3 pounds in ten days": www.freakonomics.com/blog/2005/09/18/final-guest-blog-from-seth-roberts (Molly, posted September 22, 2005), accessed January 27, 2006.

114 "Your conclusions on fructose sugar are right on the money": www.freakonomics.com/blog/ 2005/09/15/seth-roberts-on-acne-guest-blogger-part-iv (David Z., posted October 14, 2005), accessed January 4, 2006.

114 "I tried fructose water for 3–4 days and GAINED THREE POUNDS": www.freakonomics.com/blog/ 2005/09/18/final-guest-blog-from-seth-roberts (Bonnie, posted September 22, 2005), accessed January 4, 2006.

114 "I've tried the regime for about two weeks now with no results": www.freakonomics.com/blog/ 2005/09/09/freakonomics-in-the-ny-times-the-shangri-la-diet (Anonymous, posted September 30, 2005), accessed January 27, 2006.

114 "I've been on the diet for three days":

www.freakonomics.com/blog/2005/09/14/seth-roberts-guest-blogger-part-iii (Bill Q., posted September 15, 2005), accessed January 4, 2006.

115 De Benci, starting at 185 pounds: Annie's blog (many posts), accessed January 27, 2006. "that I feel I can": posted November 15, 2005.

115 Emily started at 276 pounds: Annie's blog (many posts), accessed January 27, 2006. "It is very interesting": posted November 11, 2005.

115 Julie had little luck: Annie's blog (many posts), accessed January 27, 2006. "I stopped drinking my": posted November 13, 2005.

115 Leftblanc started at 226 pounds: Annie's blog (many posts), accessed January 27, 2006.

116 Masa'il (Hendricks herself): Annie's blog (many posts), accessed January 27, 2006. "definitely irreplaceable so far": posted December 1, 2005.

116 Michelle started at 170 pounds: Annie's blog (many posts), accessed January 27, 2006. "I'm definitely making better choices": posted October 21, 2005.

116 Molly. After two weeks, she wrote: Annie's blog (many posts), accessed January 27, 2006. "Jeez, this diet makes me": posted October 1, 2005. "So much of what I": posted October 4, 2005. "I lost 12 pounds": posted December 3, 2005. "is a very useful tool": posted December 1, 2005.

117 Sarah's first post said that she had been: Annie's blog (many posts), accessed January 27, 2006.

"doing the diet for almost": posted September 29, 2005.

117 SFC started at 184 and over three months steadily lost 18 pounds: Annie's blog (many posts) accessed January 27, 2006. "This has been nearly effortless": posted November 15, 2005.

118 "Getting the real range of experiences posted": Annie's blog (Masa'il, posted November 20, 2005), accessed January 27, 2006.

118 Robert F. wrote that he had "tried the diet . . . minimal success": Annie's blog (Robert F., posted November 28, 2005), accessed January 27, 2006.

118 Agnostic wrote, "I lost 5 pounds in 3 weeks": Annie's blog (posted December 2, 2005), accessed January 27, 2006.

118 Soon after the *Freakonomics* column, www .calorielab.com . . . posted a long article about the diet: CalorieLab blog (posted September 21, 2005), accessed January 27, 2006.

119 "I am two weeks into the oil diet": CalorieLab blog/#comment-382 (Paul T., posted September 27, 2005), accessed January 4, 2006.

119 "Separating, through this diet, gimme-energy hunger": CalorieLab blog/#comment-382 (Paul T., posted October 6, 2005), accessed January 5, 2006.

119 "I am 54, 5'8" post-menopausal at 146 lbs.": CalorieLab blog/#comment-263 (Jill, posted September 29, 2005), accessed January 5, 2006.

119 "I have been using the 'Shangri-la' diet now for almost a month": CalorieLab blog/#comment-393 (Alice H., posted October 7, 2005), accessed January 5, 2006.

120 "Have been doing this for 3 weeks": CalorieLab blog/#comment-436 (David Z., posted October 14, 2005), accessed January 5, 2006.

120 "I just have to say it works. I tried it for 2 weeks": CalorieLab blog/#comment-461 (Neema, posted October 18, 2005), accessed January 5, 2006.

120 "I've been following your Shangri La guidelines now for 3 days": CalorieLab blog/#comment-695 (Carmen, posted November 18, 2005), accessed January 5, 2006.

120 "My family doctor recommended that I try this diet": CalorieLab blog/#comment-730 (Tina, posted November 22, 2005), accessed January 5, 2006.

121 "I started this diet on 9/12": CalorieLab blog/#comment-737 (Leftblanc, posted November 23, 2005), accessed January 5, 2006.

121 "Why would I avoid restaurant food?": CalorieLab blog/#comment-743 (Leftblanc, posted November 25, 2005), accessed January 5, 2006.

121 "I can't say enough about the dramatic switch in the way I feel about food": CalorieLab blog/#comment-757 (Stephen M. [Ethesis], posted November 28, 2005), accessed January 5, 2006.

122 "I'm a 52-year-old woman, 5 feet tall": CalorieLab blog/#comment-758 (Cheryl, posted November 29, 2005), accessed January 5, 2006.

122 "I have been trying the oil": CalorieLab blog
/#comment-1151 (Imtiaz, posted December 23,
2005), accessed January 5, 2006.

Chapter 7. Changing the Rest of the World

123 "I didn't know any English at all . . . for some
obscure reason I knew the word *gluttony*":
Khaled Hosseini, talk at George Mason
University, Fairfax, Virginia, September 20, 2005
(broadcast on C-Span 2) .

123 "In the year 2001 . . . a woman will have a strong
supple and splendid body all her life": Diana
Vreeland, www.fashionwindows.com/room_
service/2001/visionaire.asp, accessed November
30, 2005.

124 In 1962, a large survey found that 13 percent of
Americans were obese: Inas Rashad and
Michael Grossman, "The Economics of
Obesity," *The Public Interest* 156 (Summer
2004): 104–112.

124 In *Food Fight* . . . television, video games, personal computers, eating away from home,
snacking, and "the glorification of overeating":
Kelly D. Brownell and Katherine Battle Horgen,
Food Fight (New York: McGraw-Hill, 2004),
35–40.

125 Time spent watching TV increased by 45 per-
cent . . . TV watching increased only a little:
David M. Cutler, Edward L. Glaeser, and Jesse
M. Shapiro, "Why Have Americans Become More
Obese?" Working Paper 9446 (Washington, D.C.:

National Bureau of Economic Research, 2003). Available at www.nber.org/papers/w9446. This paper also contains measurements of overall activity that contradict the idea that the obesity epidemic was caused by declines in activity.

125 Another reason to doubt . . . low-fat diets produce little weight loss. After a year, most people have lost only a few pounds: Walter C. Willett, "Dietary Fat Plays a Major Role in Obesity: No," *Obesity Reviews* 3 (2002): 59–60.

126 From 1976 to 1996, calorie intake at breakfast, lunch, and dinner increased little, if at all; rather, there was a big increase in snacking: David M. Cutler et al., "Why Have Americans Become More Obese?" See Table 4.

127 "As much as two-thirds of the increase in adult obesity since 1980 . . . fast-food restaurants and full-service restaurants, especially the former," and Figure 7, number of restaurants: Inas Rashad, Michael Grossman, and Shin-Yi Chou, "The Super Size of America: An Economic Estimation of Body Mass Index and Obesity in Adults," Working Paper 11584 (Washington, D.C.: National Bureau of Economic Research); available at www.nber.org/papers/w11584. The values for 1962 and 1967 were computed from the U.S. Census of Business assuming that the fraction of food establishments that are restaurants (both sit-down and take-out) was the same in the 1962 and 1967 surveys as in the 1972 survey, which provided a more detailed breakdown.

127 From 1978 to 1996, calories eaten in sit-down restaurants doubled; calories eaten in fast-food restaurants tripled: David M. Cutler et al., "Why Have Americans Become More Obese?" See Table 4.

128 In a 2003 paper . . . (or, to put it another way, a great decrease in food preparation time) from 1978 to 1996: David M. Cutler et al., "Why Have Americans Become More Obese?"

130 Dr. Antonia Demas . . . how schools can persuade students to eat new foods: Interview with Antonia Demas, November 1, 2005.

133 *Totto-Chan*: Tetsuko Kuroyanagi, *Totto-Chan: The Little Girl at the Window,* Dorothy Britton, trans. (Tokyo: Kodansha International, 1982.) "First Prize . . . spinach": page 109. "Get your mothers . . . tastes good": pages 109–110. "He was right": page 110.

135 Cargill, a huge American ingredients company, recently introduced two new sweeteners: Press release, September 12, 2005; available at www.cargill.com/news/news__releases/050912 __sucromalt.htm, accessed November 30, 2005.

Appendix. The Science Behind the Theory Behind the Diet

141 "Am I the only one who thinks this diet might be an enormous hoax perpetrated by the *Freakonomics* guys?": Annie's blog (Jennifer, posted November 18, 2005), accessed December 2, 2005.

141 "I hardly believe it myself": Annie's blog (Leftblanc, posted November 23, 2005), accessed December 2, 2005.

141 "Jaws are dropping around the studio": *Good Morning America* segment, November 14, 2005.

142 Around 1950, a London researcher named G. Kennedy: G. C. Kennedy, "The Hypothalamic Control of Food Intake in Rats," *Proceedings of the Royal Society of London,* Series B, Containing Papers of a Biological Character 137 (889) (November 1950): 535–49.

143 the hormone leptin: Stephen C. Woods, Michael W. Schwartz, Denis G. Baskin, and Randy J. Seeley, "Food intake and the regulation of body weight," *Annual Review of Psychology* 51 (2000): 255–77.

145 "To me this was Newton's apple": Interview with Michel Cabanac, October 28, 2005.

146 To test this prediction, he did an experiment in which subjects lost eight pounds by eating less of their usual food: M. Cabanac, R. Duclaux, and N. H. Spector, "Sensory Feedback in Regulation of Body Weight: Is There a Ponderostat," *Nature* 229 (5280) (January 8, 1971): 125–27.

146 "This is the first time I have ever left food on a plate at a meal": www.freakonomics.com/blog/2005/09/09/freakonomics-in-the-ny-times-the-shangri-la-diet/#comments (Jnyc, posted September 18, 2005), accessed January 27, 2006.

146 "I'm able to feel full after eating about half of

what I normally eat": www.freakonomics.com/blog/2005/09/09/freakonomics-in-the-ny-times-the-shangri-la-diet/#comments (Anonymous, posted September 20, 2005), accessed January 27, 2006.

147 To see if something similar happened with weight . . . "a very flat food," a bland liquid diet: M. Cabanac and E. F. Rabe, "Influence of a Monotonous Food on Body Weight Regulation in Humans," *Physiology & Behavior* 17 (4) (October 1976): 675–78.

148 Around the same time . . . a student in Cabanac's lab named Marc Fantino . . . nutrition without any flavor at all, in other words: Marc Fantino, "Effet de l'alimentation intragastrique au long cours chez l'homme," *Journal de Physiologie* 72 (1976): 86A.

149 Maybe if the food tasted better, they would get fat more quickly, reasoned Sclafani: Interview with Anthony Sclafani, November 11, 2005.

149 This suggested that supermarket food was quite fattening . . . not just its high fat content that made it fattening: Anthony Sclafani and Deleri Springer, "Dietary Obesity in Adult Rats: Similarities to Hypothalamic and Human Obesity Syndromes," *Physiology & Behavior* 17 (1976): 461–71.

150 By accident, he had discovered that rats have a remarkable appetite for a partially digested starch: Anthony Sclafani et al., "Sex Differences

in Polysaccharide and Sugar Preferences in Rats,"
Neuroscience and Biobehavioral Reviews 11 (2)
(Summer 1987): 241–51.

150 Sclafani and a colleague set up an apparatus . . .
directly into a rat's stomach whenever it drank:
Anthony Sclafani and Jeffrey W. Nissenbaum,
"Robust Conditioned Flavor Preference
Produced by Intragastric Starch Infusions in
Rats," *American Journal of Physiology—
Regulatory, and Integrative Comparative
Physiology*, 24 (1998): R672–R675.

151 In the following years, Sclafani and his col-
leagues did hundreds of experiments about
flavor-calorie learning: Anthony Sclafani, "How
Food Preferences Are Learned: Laboratory
Animal Models," *Proceedings of the Nutrition
Society* 54 (1995): 419–27.

152 He did so much great work . . . about whether
sugar causes obesity: Interview with Israel
Ramirez, October 27, 2005.

152 "It is widely believed," the paper began, "that
consumption of sucrose may predispose human
beings to obesity": Israel Ramirez, "When Does
Sucrose Increase Appetite and Adiposity?"
Appetite 9 (1987): 1–19.

154 The right amount of water could *double* the rats'
weight gain: Israel Ramirez, "Diet Texture,
Moisture and Starch Type in Dietary Obesity,"
Physiology & Behavior 41 (1987): 149–54.

155 Maybe the saccharin would make the food taste

better so the animals would eat more of it: Israel Ramirez, "Stimulation of Energy Intake and Growth by Saccharin in Rats," *Journal of Nutrition* 120 (1990): 123–33. "First evidence": page 132.

INDEX

Page numbers in *italic* indicate figures;
those in **bold** indicate tables.

ABOUT THE AUTHOR

Seth Roberts, Ph.D., is a professor of psychology at the University of California at Berkeley. He serves on the editorial advisory board of the journal *Nutrition* and has published dozens of scientific articles on many topics, including health, nutrition, and weight control. His work has appeared in major scientific journals such as *The Lancet* and *Behavioral and Brain Sciences.* Articles about his work have appeared in the *New York Times* and *Harper's.* Roberts lives in Berkeley, California.